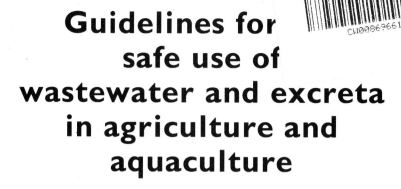

Guidelines for safe use of wastewater and excreta in agriculture and aquaculture

Measures for public health protection

Prepared by
Duncan Mara
University of Leeds,
Leeds, England
&
Sandy Cairncross
London School of Hygiene and Tropical Medicine
London, England

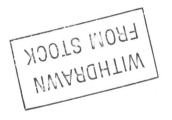

World Health Organization
Geneva 1989

ISBN 92 4 154248 9

TYPESET IN INDIA
PRINTED IN ENGLAND

88/7837-Macmillan/Clays-5000

Contents

Foreword

These Guidelines form the main output of a project on health hazards of reuse of waste, which has been executed by the World Health Organization and financed by the United Nations Environment Programme. The overall objective of the project and of these Guidelines is to encourage the safe use of treated wastewater and excreta-derived products for agriculture and aquaculture in such a way as to protect the health of workers and consumers.

The Guidelines are intended for planners and decision-makers in Ministries of Health, Water and Agriculture and other government agencies and for consulting engineers concerned with the use of wastewater and excreta-derived products for agriculture and aquaculture. The guidance provided is aimed at controlling the transmission of communicable diseases. The discussion of health risks is thus limited to microbiological contamination, and chemical pollution is not included.

The suggested quality criteria for the safe use of wastewater in agriculture and aquaculture consist of a re-evaluation of the guidelines proposed by a group of experts in 1973 (WHO Technical Report Series, No. 517). Progress in applied research and wider experience in a number of countries have shown that limits on the presence of viable ova of parasitic helminths are necessary to safeguard public health. On the other hand, it has also been shown that the quality criterion for faecal coliforms could be relaxed without creating an unacceptable risk to the exposed population. Revised quality criteria are based on epidemiological evidence of actual risks to public health, rather than on potential hazards indicated by the survival of pathogens on crops and in soil.

These Guidelines were prepared by Professor Duncan Mara, University of Leeds, and Dr Sandy Cairncross, London School of Hygiene and Tropical Medicine. The case materials presented in the document are largely based on reports from Dr Martin Strauss, International Reference Centre for Waste Disposal, Dübendorf, and Dr Ursula Blumenthal, London School of Hygiene and Tropical Medicine; from World Bank Technical Paper No. 51, "Wastewater irrigation in developing countries: health effects and technical solutions", by Professor Hillel Shuval and colleagues at the Hebrew University of Jerusalem; and from the proceedings of the FAO Seminar on "Treatment and reuse of sewage effluents for irrigation" held in Cyprus in 1985.

The draft Guidelines were reviewed by a group of experts at the Second Project Meeting on the Safe Use of Human Wastes in Agriculture and Aquaculture in Adelboden, Switzerland, in June 1987. The meeting was organized by the International Reference Centre for Waste Disposal and WHO with financial support from the United Nations Environment Programme. The participants in the meeting are listed below.

Participants

Dr Bakir Abisudjak Panjadjaran University, Bandung, Indonesia.

Dr Humberto Romero-Alvarez Secretariat of Agriculture and Hydraulic Resources, Mexico City, Mexico.

Dr Abdullah Arar Food and Agriculture Organization of the United Nations, Rome, Italy.

Mr Sadok Attallah Ministry of Public Health, Tunis, Tunisia.

Dr Carl Bartone World Bank, Washington, DC, USA.

Dr Eduardo Bauer Water Supply and Sanitation Service, Lima, Peru.

Dr Asit Biswas International Society for Ecological Modelling, Oxford, England.

Dr Ursula Blumenthal London School of Hygiene and Tropical Medicine, London, England.

Dr Armando Caceres Centre for Mesoamerican Studies on Appropriate Technology, Guatemala City, Guatemala.

Dr Sandy Cairncross London School of Hygiene and Tropical Medicine, London, England.

Dr Paul Guo WHO Western Pacific Regional Centre for the Promotion of Environmental Planning and Applied Studies, Kuala Lumpur, Malaysia.

Dr Ivanildo Hespanhol World Health Organization, Geneva, Switzerland.

Mr John Kalbermatten Kalbermatten Associates, Washington, DC, USA.

Professor Duncan Mara University of Leeds, Leeds, England.

Professor Warren Pescod University of Newcastle-upon-Tyne, Newcastle-upon-Tyne, England.

Ms Silvie Peter International Reference Centre for Waste Disposal, Dübendorf, Switzerland.

Dr André Prost World Health Organization, Geneva, Switzerland.

Dr Alex Redekopp International Development Research Centre, Ottawa, Canada.

Dr Roland Schertenlieb (*Chairman*) International Reference Centre for Waste Disposal, Dübendorf, Switzerland.

Dr Donald Sharp International Development Research Centre, Ottawa, Canada.

Professor Hillel Shuval Hebrew University of Jerusalem, Jerusalem, Israel.

Dr Martin Strauss International Reference Centre for Waste Disposal, Dübendorf, Switzerland.

**Guidelines for the safe use of wastewater and
excreta in agriculture and aquaculture:**
Measures for public health protection

Executive Summary

Introduction

The overall objective of these Guidelines is to encourage the safe use
of wastewater and excreta in agriculture and aquaculture in a manner
that protects the health of the workers involved and of the public at
large. In this context "wastewater" refers to domestic sewage and
municipal wastewaters that do not contain substantial quantities of
industrial effluent; "excreta" refers to nightsoil and to excreta-
derived products such as sludge and septage. Health protection
considerations will generally require that some treatment be applied
to these wastes to remove pathogenic organisms. Other health
protection measures are also considered, including crop restriction,
waste application techniques and human exposure control.

The Guidelines are addressed primarily to senior professionals in
the various sectors relevant to wastes reuse, and aim to prevent
transmission of communicable diseases while optimizing resource
conservation and waste recycling. Emphasis is therefore on control
of microbiological contamination rather than on avoidance of the
health hazards of chemical pollution, which is of only minor importance in the reuse of domestic wastes and is adequately covered in
other publications. Purely agricultural aspects are considered only in
so far as they are relevant to health protection.

Hygiene standards applied to wastes reuse in the past, based solely
on potential pathogen survival, have been stricter than necessary. A
meeting of sanitary engineers, epidemiologists and social scientists,
convened by the World Health Organization, the World Bank and
the International Reference Centre for Waste Disposal and held in
Engelberg, Switzerland, in 1985, proposed a more realistic approach
to the use of treated wastewater and excreta, based on the best and
most recent epidemiological evidence. The recommendations of
the resulting Engelberg Report have formed the basis for these
Guidelines.

Scope

Sections 2 and 3 of the Guidelines review the history and benefits of wastes reuse and cite examples of existing practices in various parts of the world. Public health aspects, including the practical implications of recent epidemiological advances, are introduced in Section 4, and sociocultural factors are considered in Section 5. Section 6 discusses environmental protection and enhancement through wastes reuse. Feasible and appropriate control measures for public health protection are comprehensively reviewed in Section 7, and the institutional, legal and financial aspects of project planning and implementation are discussed in Section 8.

Human wastes as a resource

Human wastes are a widely used resource in many parts of the world. The Guidelines concentrate on the following three practices, which are the most common:

- use of wastewater for crop irrigation;

- use of excreta for soil fertilization and soil structure improvement;

- use of wastewater and excreta in aquaculture.

Wastewater use in agriculture

In the past two decades there has been a notable increase in the use of wastewater for crop irrigation, especially in arid and seasonally arid areas of both industrialized and developing countries. This has occurred as a result of several factors:

- the increasing scarcity of alternative waters for irrigation, exacerbated by increasing urban demand for potable water supplies, and the growing recognition by water resource planners of the importance and value of wastewater reuse;

- the high cost of artificial fertilizers and the recognition of the value of nutrients in wastewater, which significantly increase crop yield;

- the demonstration that health risks and soil damage are minimal if the necessary precautions are taken;

- the high cost of advanced wastewater treatment plants; and

- the sociocultural acceptance of the practice.

Normal domestic and municipal wastewater is composed of 99% water and 0.1% suspended, colloidal and dissolved solids — organic and inorganic compounds, including macronutrients such as nitrogen, phosphorus and potassium as well as essential micronutrients. Industrial effluents may add toxic compounds, but not in detrimental quantities, and only the boron sensitivity of the crop being irrigated needs consideration. The application rate of wastewater is calculated in the same way as for freshwater irrigation, with due regard to evapotranspiration demand, leaching requirements and salinity and sodicity control.

Excreta use in agriculture

The ancient practice of applying human excreta to the land has maintained soil fertility in many countries of Eastern Asia and the Western Pacific for over 4000 years, and remains the only agricultural use option in areas without sewerage facilities. Most households in developing countries will continue to lack sewerage systems in the foreseeable future; emphasis should therefore be placed on establishing on-site sanitation systems that readily permit the safe use of stored excreta — for example, alternating twin-pit or pour-flush latrines and compost toilets.

Each person typically produces 1.8 litres of excreta daily; this comprises 350 grams of dry solids, including 90 grams of organic matter, 20 grams of nitrogen, plus other nutrients — mainly phosphorus and potassium. Excreta treatment not only destroys pathogenic microorganisms but also converts these nutrients to forms more readily usable by crops and stabilizes the organic matter, producing a better soil conditioner. Excreta and excreta-derived products are generally applied to the land before planting at annual rates of 5–30 tonnes per hectare (t/ha) (10 t/ha = 1 kg/m^2).

Excreta and wastewater use in aquaculture

Aquaculture refers to the ancient practices of fish culture, notably of carp and tilapia, and the growing of aquatic crops, such as water spinach, water chestnut, water calthrop and lotus. Fertilization of aquaculture ponds with human and animal wastes has been practised for thousands of years in Asia; today at least two-thirds of the world yield of farmed fish comes from ponds fertilized in this way. China produces 60% of the world's farmed fish in only 27% of the world's area of fish-ponds; the mean annual yield from Chinese fish-ponds is 3200 kg/ha but well managed intensive polyculture ponds can produce up to 7000 kg/ha. Such fish represent the cheapest source of animal protein.

Fish can also be successfully farmed in the maturation ponds of a series of waste stabilization ponds: annual yields of up to 3000 kg/ha have been obtained. The sale of the harvested fish can be used to pay for improved operation and maintenance of municipal sewerage systems.

Examples of human waste reuse

Of the many examples of human wastes reuse, the few described in the Guidelines were chosen to represent a wide range of locations and sociocultural settings, scales of operation, treatment processes, application techniques and crops harvested. The examples given are:

Wastewater use in agriculture: Australia, Federal Republic of Germany, India, Mexico, Tunisia.

Excreta use in agriculture: China, Guatemala, India, United States of America.

Wastewater and excreta use in aquaculture: India, Indonesia.

Public health aspects

Health risks

Excreta-related diseases are very common in developing countries, and excreta and wastewater contain correspondingly high concentrations of excreted pathogens — bacteria, viruses, protozoa and helminths. About 30 such diseases are of public health importance, and many of these are of specific importance in waste reuse schemes. However, the agricultural or aquacultural use of excreta and wastewater can result in an *actual* risk to public health only if *all* of the following occur:

(a) *either* an infective dose of an excreted pathogen reaches a field or pond, *or* the pathogen multiplies in the field or pond to form an infective dose;

(b) the infective dose reaches a human host;

(c) the host becomes infected; and

(d) the infection causes disease or further transmission.

If (d) does not occur, then (a), (b) and (c) can pose only *potential* risks to public health. Moreover, if this sequence of events is broken at any point, the potential risks cannot combine to constitute an actual risk.

It is now possible to design and implement schemes for human wastes reuse that pose no risk to public health, but this requires an understanding of the epidemiology of the infections in relation to wastes reuse. In this way, adequate standards for the microbiological quality of excreta and wastewater intended for reuse can be established and public health properly protected.

Epidemiological evidence

The actual public health importance of excreta or wastewater reuse can be assessed only by an epidemiological study of the particular practice to determine whether it results in measurably greater incidence or prevalence of disease, or intensity of infection, than occurs in its absence. Such studies are methodologically difficult, and there have been only a few well designed epidemiological studies on human wastes reuse; more evidence is available about wastewater irrigation than about excreta use in agriculture or about aquacultural use.

Wastewater irrigation. A recent World Bank report (Technical Paper No. 51) reviewed all available epidemiological studies on wastewater irrigation and concluded that:

• Crop irrigation with untreated wastewater causes significant excess intestinal nematode infection in crop consumers and field workers. Field workers, especially those who work barefoot, are likely to have more intense infections, particularly with hookworms, than those not working in wastewater-irrigated fields.

• Irrigation with adequately treated wastewater does not lead to excess intestinal nematode infection in field workers or crop consumers.

5

- Cholera, and probably typhoid, can be effectively transmitted by irrigation of vegetable crops with untreated wastewater.

- Cattle grazing on pasture irrigated with raw wastewater may become infected with beef tapeworm, but there is little evidence of actual risks to humans.

- There is limited evidence that the health of people living near fields irrigated with raw wastewater is negatively affected, either directly by contact with the soil or indirectly by contact with farm workers. In communities with high standards of personal hygiene any negative effects are generally restricted to an excess incidence of benign, often viral, gastroenteritis, although there may also be an excess of bacterial infections.

- Sprinkler irrigation with treated wastewater may promote aerosol transmission of excreted viruses, but this is likely to be rare in practice because most people have normally high levels of immunity to endemic viral diseases.

It is clear that, when *untreated* wastewater is used to irrigate crops, there is a high actual health risk from intestinal nematodes and bacteria but little or no risk from viruses. Thus, treatment of wastewater is a highly effective method of safeguarding public health.

Excreta use in agriculture. A recent report (No. 05/85) published by the International Reference Centre for Waste Disposal reviewed epidemiological evidence on the agricultural use of excreta and concluded that:

- Crop fertilization with untreated excreta causes significant excess intestinal nematode infection in crop consumers and field workers.

- There is evidence that excreta treatment can reduce the transmission of nematode infection.

- Excreta fertilization of rice paddies may lead to excess schistosomiasis infection among rice farmers.

- Cattle may become infected with tapeworm but are unlikely to contract salmonellosis.

Aquacultural use. The IRCWD report also reviewed evidence for disease transmission associated with aquacultural use of excreta and wastewater; its findings were less conclusive than those concerning agricultural use because of the limited quantity and quality of available data.

Clear epidemiological evidence exists for the transmission of certain trematode diseases, principally those caused by *Clonorchis* (oriental liver fluke) and *Fasciolopsis* (giant intestinal fluke), but not for transmission of schistosomiasis (bilharzia), which is none the less a major potential risk to those who work in excreta-fertilized ponds. There was no conclusive evidence for bacterial disease transmission by passive transference of the pathogens by fish and aquatic vegetables, although this too remains a potential risk.

Microbiological quality criteria

Experts attending the First Project Meeting on the Safe Use of Human Wastes in Agriculture and Aquaculture, in Engelberg, Switzerland, in 1985, reviewed epidemiological evidence concerning the agricultural use of human wastes and formulated the Engelberg Guidelines for the microbiological quality of *treated* wastewater intended for crop irrigation. Those guidelines recommend that treated wastewater should contain:

• <1 viable intestinal nematode egg per litre (on an arithmetic mean basis) for restricted or unrestricted irrigation; and

• <1000 faecal coliform bacteria per 100 millilitres (on a geometric mean basis) for unrestricted irrigation.

Unrestricted irrigation refers to irrigation of trees, fodder and industrial crops, fruit trees and pasture, and restricted irrigation to irrigation of edible crops, sports fields and public parks.

The guidelines are also applicable to agricultural use if the excreta, in the form of liquid nightsoil for example, is applied to the field while crops are growing.

The intestinal nematode egg guideline value is designed to protect the health of both field workers and crop consumers and represents a high degree of egg removal from the wastewater (>99%). The faecal coliform guideline value is less stringent than earlier recommendations, but is in accord with modern standards for bathing waters, for example, and more than adequate to protect the health of consumers. Effluents complying with both guideline values can be simply and

7

reliably produced by treatment in a well designed series of waste stabilization ponds.

Guidelines for the microbiological quality of treated excreta and wastewater for aquacultural use were developed at the Second Project Meeting held in Adelboden, Switzerland, in June 1987. These recommend zero viable trematode eggs per litre or per kilogram (on an arithmetic mean basis), and less than 10 000 faecal coliform bacteria per 100 millilitres or 100 grams (on a geometric mean basis). Such a stringent trematode guideline is necessary as these pathogens multiply very greatly in their first intermediate aquatic host. The value for faecal coliforms assumes a 90% reduction of these bacteria in the pond, so that fish and aquatic vegetables are not exposed to more than 1000 faecal coliforms per 100 millilitres.

Sociocultural aspects

Human behavioural patterns are a key determinant in the transmission of excreta-related diseases. The social feasibility of changing certain behavioural patterns in order to introduce excreta or wastewater use schemes, or to reduce disease transmission in existing schemes, can be assessed only with a prior understanding of the cultural significance of practices that appear to be social preferences yet which facilitate disease transmission. Cultural beliefs vary so widely in different parts of the world that it is not possible to assume that excreta or wastewater use practices that have evolved in one area can readily be transferred to another. A thorough assessment of the local sociocultural context is always necessary during the project planning stage, otherwise the project may be confidently expected to fail.

Environmental aspects

Properly planned and managed excreta and wastewater use schemes can have a positive environmental impact, as well as increasing agricultural and aquacultural yields. Environmental improvement results from several factors, including:

- Avoidance of surface water pollution, which occurs if unused wastewaters are discharged into rivers or lakes. Major pollution problems such as dissolved oxygen depletion, eutrophication, foaming and fish kills can be avoided.

- Conservation or more rational usage of freshwater resources, especially in arid and semi-arid areas: fresh water for urban demand, wastewater for agriculture.

- Reduced requirements for artificial fertilizers, with a concomitant reduction in energy expenditure and industrial pollution elsewhere.

- Soil conservation through humus build-up and prevention of land erosion.

- Desertification control and desert reclamation through irrigation and fertilization of tree belts.

- Improved urban amenity through irrigation and fertilization of green spaces for recreation and visual appeal.

Soil and groundwater pollution are potential disadvantages of the agricultural use of excreta and wastewater which can be minimized by scientifically sound planning and effective management of irrigation and fertilization regimes.

Technical options for health protection

Available measures for health protection can be grouped under four main headings:

- treatment of waste;

- crop restriction;

- waste application methods;

- control of human exposure.

It will often be desirable to apply a combination of several methods. The technical factors affecting each option are considered.

Waste treatment

The degree of pathogen removal by a waste treatment process is best expressed in terms of $\log_{10}$ units. The Engelberg quality guideline for unrestricted irrigation requires a bacterial reduction of at least

4 log units and a helminth egg removal of 3 log units. Helminth removal alone is sufficient to protect field workers. A lesser degree of removal can be considered if other health protection measures are envisaged or if the quality will be further improved after treatment. This can occur by dilution in naturally occurring water, by prolonged storage or by transport over long distances in a river or canal.

Without supplementary disinfection, conventional processes (plain sedimentation, activated sludge, biofiltration, aerated lagoons and oxidation ditches) cannot produce an effluent that complies with the Engelberg guideline for unrestricted irrigation. Moreover, conventional wastewater treatment systems are not generally effective for helminth egg removal.

Waste stabilization ponds are usually the wastewater treatment method of choice in warm climates. A series of ponds with a total retention time of about 11 days can be designed to achieve adequate helminth removal; depending on temperature, about twice that time is usually required to reach the bacterial guideline. The high degree of confidence with which pond series can meet the Engelberg guidelines is only one of their many advantages: others are low cost and simple operation. The only disadvantage of pond systems is the relatively large area of land required.

Disinfection — usually chlorination — of raw sewage has never been fully achieved in practice, but it will reduce the numbers of excreted bacteria in the effluent from a conventional treatment plant. However, a high, uniform and predictable level of disinfection efficiency is extremely difficult to maintain, and chlorination also leaves most helminth eggs unharmed.

Another problem is the cost of chlorine. A more appropriate treatment option is to add one or more ponds in series to a conventional treatment plant. The addition of polishing ponds is a suitable measure to upgrade an existing wastewater treatment plant.

Excreta treatment is not required for excreta applied to the land by sub-surface injection or placed in trenches before the start of the growing season. To achieve the guideline for helminthic quality, excreta must be stored for at least a year at ambient temperatures; alternatively, nightsoil and septage can be directly treated in waste stabilization ponds.

Heat treatment of excreta. Two methods of treating excreta at high temperatures may be used to reduce the minimum 12-month storage period needed to reach the Engelberg standard:

- batch thermophilic digestion at 50 °C for 13 days;

- forced aeration composting.

From the agricultural viewpoint composting has several advantages.

Crop restriction

Agriculture. If the Engelberg standard is not fully met, it may still be possible to grow selected crops without risk to the consumer. Crops can be broadly categorized according to the required extent of health protection measures:

Category A—Protection needed only for field workers. Includes industrial crops such as cotton, sisal, grains and forestry, as well as food crops for canning.

Category B—Further measures may be needed. Applies to pasture, green fodder and tree crops and to fruit and vegetables that are peeled or cooked before eating.

Category C—Treatment to Engelberg "unrestricted" guidelines essential. Covers fresh vegetables, spray-irrigated fruit, and parks, lawns and golf courses.

Irrigation limited to certain crops and conditions, such as Category A, is commonly referred to as restricted irrigation.

Crop restriction provides protection to consumers but not to farm workers and their families. It should be complemented by other measures, such as partial waste treatment, controlled waste application or human exposure control. Partial treatment to the helminthic part of the Engelberg quality guideline would protect the health of field workers in most settings and is cheaper than full treatment.

Crop restriction is feasible and is facilitated in several circumstances, including the following:

- where a law-abiding society or strong law enforcement exists;

- where a public body controls allocation of the wastes;

- where an irrigation project has strong central management;

- where there is adequate demand for the crops allowed under crop restriction and where they fetch a reasonable price;

- where there is little market pressure in favour of excluded crops (such as those in Category C).

Application of wastewater and excreta

Wastewater in agriculture. Irrigation water, including treated wastewater, can be applied to the land in the following five ways:

- by flooding (border irrigation), wetting almost all the land surface;

- by furrows, wetting only part of the ground surface;

- by sprinklers, in which the soil is wetted in much the same way as by rain;

- by subsurface irrigation, in which the surface is wetted little but the subsoil is saturated;

- by localized (trickle, drip or bubbler) irrigation, in which water is applied at each individual plant at an adjustable rate.

Flooding involves the least investment but probably the greatest risk to field workers.

If the water is not of Engelberg bacterial quality but is required for use on Category B crops, sprinkler irrigation should not be used except for pasture or fodder crops, and border irrigation should not be used for vegetables.

Subsurface irrigation can give the greatest degree of health protection as well as using water more efficiently and often producing higher yields. However, it is expensive and a high degree of reliable treatment is needed to prevent clogging of the small holes (emitters) through which water is slowly released into the soil. Bubbler irrigation, developed for localized irrigation of trees, avoids the need for emitters to regulate the flow to each tree.

Excreta in agriculture. Untreated or insufficiently treated excreta should be applied to land only by placing it in covered trenches before the start of the growing season, or by subsurface injection using specialized equipment. Nightsoil treated only to the helminthic quality guideline may pose a greater risk to field workers than restricted irrigation with wastewater; the risk can be minimized only by exposure control measures.

Aquaculture. Keeping fish in clean water for at least 2 to 3 weeks before harvest will remove any residual objectionable odours and reduce contamination with faecal microorganisms. However, such depuration does not guarantee complete removal of pathogens from fish tissues and digestive tracts unless the contamination is very slight.

Human exposure control

Agriculture. Four groups of people can be identified as being at potential risk from the agricultural use of wastewater and excreta:

- agricultural field workers and their families;

- crop handlers;

- consumers (of crops, meat and milk);

- those living near the affected fields.

Exposure of field workers to hookworm infection can be reduced by continuous in-field use of appropriate footwear, but this may be quite difficult to achieve.

Immunization against helminthic infections and most diarrhoeal diseases is not feasible, but it may be worth immunizing highly exposed groups against typhoid and hepatitis A. Additional protection may be afforded by adequate medical facilities, by regular chemotherapeutic control of intense nematode infections in children, and by control of anaemia. Chemotherapy and immunization cannot be considered an adequate strategy but could be beneficial as temporary palliative measures.

Risks to consumers can be reduced by thorough cooking and by high standards of hygiene. Tapeworm transmission can be controlled by meat inspection.

Local residents should be fully informed of the location of all fields where human wastes are used so that they and their children may avoid them. There is no evidence that those living near wastewater-irrigated fields are at significant risk from sprinkler irrigation schemes, but sprinklers should not be used within 50–100 m of houses or roads.

Aquaculture. Schistosomiasis is best controlled by treatment and snail control. Regular chemotherapy would be beneficial in endemic areas. Local residents should be informed which ponds are fertilized with wastes. Provision of adequate sanitation and clean water supplies is also an important factor in limiting human exposure.

Planning and implementation

Resources planning

The use of wastewater and excreta touches the responsibilities of several ministries or agencies. The active participation of the Health and Agriculture Ministries is especially necessary. It is usually advantageous to establish an interagency committee or possibly a separate parastatal organization to be responsible for the sector, whose first task, as an integral part of water resources planning, is to establish a national plan for wastes reuse. This will normally include plans to improve existing reuse practices as well as to implement new reuse projects.

Improvement of existing practices

The use of human wastes for crop and fish production often takes place illegally and without official recognition by the health authorities. Banning the practice is unlikely to reduce either its prevalence or the public health risk involved, and may make it more difficult than ever to supervise and control. A more promising approach is to provide support to improve existing use practices, not only to minimize health risks but also to increase productivity.

Some legal control will usually be required, although it is easier to make regulations than to enforce them. Measures to protect public health are particularly difficult to implement when there are many individual sources or owners of the waste. The measures required to bring the waste under unified control will often entail setting up new schemes.

The first stage in any attempt to improve existing practices must be a diligent effort to identify them, combined with tactful and informal conversations with farmers, local officials and interested local bodies. Where an existing practice contravenes regulations, it is important to investigate why those regulations are not being enforced: possible reasons range from inappropriate standards to lack of resources for enforcement.

Policy options

The following sections consider the feasibility, planning and implementation of the available options.

(a) Treatment

Wastewater. Treatment is difficult to implement when wastewater comes from a variety of sources, such as overflowing septic tanks. One approach may be to take action against those who produce the wastewater, to prevent the environmental pollution it causes. In other cases, the only solution may be to build a sewer system and sewage treatment works.

Excreta. Treatment is much more readily implemented where a single body such as a municipality collects or at least treats the excreta. Local demonstration plots may persuade individual farmers to treat excreta, by showing that crop yields are increased. This is a job for the agricultural extension service.

Aquaculture. One treatment option for aquaculture is to connect ponds in series (or to divide one pond into compartments connected in series), and avoid harvesting from the first pond. It may be necessary to establish cooperative arrangements between the owners of the different ponds.

(b) Crop restriction

The enforcement of crop restrictions on a large number of small farmers can be difficult but not impossible. In some countries, the existing agricultural planning machinery allows firm control of all crops grown. However, where there is no local experience, the feasibility of crop restrictions should first be tested in a trial area. Arrangements are needed for marketing permitted crops, as well as for assisted access to agricultural credit.

(c) Application

A change in irrigation method to reduce health risks is most needed when the current practice is flooding. Farmers may need help with preparing the land to make other methods possible. Arguments that may persuade them to change include the greater efficiency of other irrigation methods and reduced mosquito nuisance. If the agricultural extension service is not able to promote hygienic application methods, the body controlling waste distribution may still be able to do so.

(d) Human exposure control

Measures to reduce exposure to diarrhoeal diseases generally and to promote good case management are well known components of primary health care. Obvious measures are provision of adequate water supplies and sanitation facilities. Care is required to ensure that the wastes do not contaminate nearby sources of drinking-water.

Where salaried field or pond workers are involved, employers' responsibilities are often set down in existing legislation on occupational health. Hygiene education is also needed for crop handlers and consumers; markets may be the ideal places for advising consumers on this subject.

Once the necessary precautions have been explained, local residents are best placed to ensure that their health is not jeopardized. A residents' health committee can be a focus for a health education campaign as well as monitoring the practice of wastes reuse.

Treatment of agricultural workers and their families for intestinal helminth infections is relatively easy to administer in a formal wastewater irrigation scheme, although additional health personnel may be required. Where wastewater is used on many small farms, the identification and treatment of exposed persons may become quite expensive, so that mass chemotherapy then becomes preferable to the selective treatment of individuals.

New schemes

Upgrading of existing schemes may be needed to improve productivity or to reduce health risks and should generally take priority over developing new schemes. Attention should be paid not only to the technical improvements required but also to the need for better management of schemes and to their improved operation and maintenance.

A pilot project is particularly necessary in countries with little or no experience of the planned use of excreta or wastewater. The problem of health protection is only one of a number of interconnected questions that are difficult to answer without local experience of the kind a pilot project can give. A pilot project should operate for at least one growing season and may then be translated into a demonstration project with training facilities for local operators and farmers.

Project planning

In many respects, planning requirements for excreta and wastewater use are similar to those for any other irrigation and fertilization schemes. For each scheme, the planner should seek to maximize benefits in a manner consistent with the need to protect health and minimize costs. Assessing the benefits requires a forecast not only of crop yields but also of prices. This in turn demands a survey to establish that an adequate market exists for the crops.

For the plan to be useful it must take account of the time-scale. A 20-year planning horizon is often considered for irrigation projects, with a modest beginning followed by phased expansion. Wastewater projects will be affected by progressive change in the quantity and quality of wastewater available.

The organizational pattern of a wastes reuse scheme will be determined largely by the existing land use patterns and institutions. Farmers need security of tenure of their land and of their right to the wastewater, especially if they are to make capital investments or change to new crops.

Large schemes need a full-time professional management staff, preferably under a single agency. Issuing and renewing permits for use of the resource can be made conditional on the observance of sanitary practices. It is common to deal with the farmers or pond owners through users' associations, giving them the task of enforcing the regulations that must be complied with for a permit to be renewed.

A joint committee or management board, which may include representatives of these associations, as well as of any particularly large users, of the authorities that collect and distribute the wastes and of the local health authorities, has proved its worth in many schemes.

Various support services to farmers are relevant to health protection and should be considered at the planning stage. They include the supply of farm machinery, agricultural credit, marketing services, primary health care and training. It is often necessary to begin training programmes before the start of the project. Similarly, the likely need for extension services must be estimated, and provision made for them to be available to farmers after implementation.

Legislation

The introduction or promotion of new projects for agricultural or aquacultural use of wastewater or excreta may require legislative action. Five areas deserve attention:

- creation of new institutions or allocation of new powers to existing bodies;

- roles of and relationships between national and local government in the sector;

- rights of access to and ownership of the wastes, including public regulation of their use;

- land tenure;

- public health and agricultural legislation: waste quality standards, crop restrictions, application methods, occupational health, food hygiene, etc.

Economic and financial considerations

Economic appraisal considers whether a project is worthwhile; financial planning looks at how projects are to be paid for. Improvements to existing practices also require some financial planning.

Economic appraisal. The economic appraisal of wastewater irrigation schemes must compare them with the alternative—what would be done in the absence of the scheme. The cost of the wastewater includes the cost of any additional treatment required, of conveying it to the field and of applying it to the crop. However, it is essential to subtract from this the cost of the alternative arrangements for wastewater disposal if the project were not implemented. The economic appraisal of excreta use and aquacultural schemes is less sophisticated, as some of the benefits are more difficult to quantify.

Financial planning. A charge is normally levied for distributing the waste to farmers, the level of which must be decided at the planning stage. A farmer will pay for wastewater for irrigation only if its cost is less than that of the cheapest alternative water and the value of the nutrients it contains. In the case of aquaculture and the use of excreta, the price is usually based on the marginal cost of treating and conveying the wastes or on the value of their nutrient content, whichever is the lower.

It is not always appropriate or feasible to meet the cost of health protection by charging for the use of the wastes. Financial considerations regarding each of the four types of health protection measure are discussed below.

(a) **Treatment.** The costs of treatment are usually justified on grounds of environmental pollution control. However, the treatment of wastes to a quality adequate for use in agriculture may involve additional costs, some of which can be met by the sale of the treated wastes. If individual farmers are to be encouraged to treat nightsoil or wastewater, they may need credit to help with the capital cost of any construction required.

(b) **Crop restriction.** Crop restriction may mean that less need be spent on treatment, but if adequate financial provision is not made for its enforcement it will not be effective.

(c) **Application.** Since preparation of the fields helps farmers avoid other expenditure, the cost can be recovered from them in the same way as other irrigation costs. Localized irrigation uses less water and can produce higher yields, and farmers may find it worth while to change to this method in some circumstances.

(d) **Human exposure control.** Protective clothing will normally be paid for by the workers who wear it or by their employers. The cost of chemotherapy is likely to be borne by the health service.

Monitoring and evaluation

Health protection measures require regular monitoring to ensure their continued effectiveness. Arrangements must be made for feedback of information to those who implement the health protection measures and for enforcement of the measures where necessary. Appropriate aspects for regular monitoring and evaluation include the following:

• **Implementation of the measures themselves.** This can be monitored by simple surveys.

- **Wastes quality.** It may be more fruitful to monitor the functioning of the treatment system than to take frequent samples for
- analysis. The Engelberg guideline values are intended not as standards for quality surveillance but as design goals for use in planning a treatment system. The lack of laboratory capacity for monitoring quality is not an adequate reason for not using wastes.

- **Crop quality.** Microbiological monitoring of crops is the task of the Ministry of Health as enforcer of public health regulations.

- **Disease surveillance.** This should focus upon farm workers. The minimum for any scheme is regular stool survey of a sample of workers for intestinal parasites. Where typhoid is endemic, a serological survey can be carried out at the same time.

I
Introduction

I.I Objectives

The overall objective of these Guidelines is to encourage the safe use of wastewater and excreta in agriculture and aquaculture, in such a manner as to protect the health of both the workers involved and the public at large. In the context of these Guidelines "wastewater" refers to domestic sewage and municipal wastewaters which do not contain substantial quantities of industrial effluent; "excreta" refers not only to nightsoil, but also to excreta-derived products such as sludge and septage.[1] Health protection needs will generally require that these wastes be used after some treatment to remove pathogenic organisms. Consideration is also given to other methods of health protection, for example crop restriction, appropriate waste application techniques, and human exposure control.

These Guidelines are addressed primarily to senior professionals in the various sectors relevant to wastes reuse, including planning, public health, sanitary engineering, water resources, and agriculture and fisheries. The guidance given is aimed at preventing communicable disease transmission while optimizing resource conservation and recycling. Emphasis is thus directed towards the control of microbiological contamination rather than the avoidance of health hazards caused by chemical pollutants, since these are of only minor importance in the reuse of domestic wastes and are in any case adequately covered in other publications.[2] Similarly, purely agricultural aspects are considered only in so far as they are relevant to health protection.

Recent advances in epidemiology have shown that past standards for hygiene in wastes reuse, which were based solely on potential pathogen survival, are stricter than is necessary to avoid health risks. A meeting of sanitary engineers, epidemiologists and social scientists, convened by the World Health Organization, the World Bank and the International Reference Centre for Waste Disposal and held in Engelberg, Switzerland in 1985, proposed a more realistic

---

[1] For a definition of these and other technical terms, see Glossary, page 184.
[2] See Bibliography, page 183.

approach to the use of treated wastewater and excreta based on the best available epidemiological evidence, which has been comprehensively reviewed by Shuval et al. (1986) and Blum & Feachem (1985). The Engelberg Report recommendations (IRCWD, 1985) have formed the basis for the general approach to public health protection adopted in these Guidelines.

1.2 Scope

Sections 2 and 3 of the Guidelines provide an overview of the history and benefits of wastes reuse, together with some examples of existing practices in various parts of the world. An introduction to public health aspects, including the practical implications of recent epidemiological advances, is given in Section 4, and sociocultural factors are considered in Section 5. Environmental protection and enhancement through wastes reuse are discussed in Section 6.

A comprehensive review of the feasible and appropriate control measures for public health protection is given in Section 7. The institutional, legal and financial aspects of project planning and implementation are discussed in Section 8, having regard to the various steps necessary to ensure that human wastes are used to their maximum advantage in agriculture and aquaculture without endangering public health.

2

Human wastes as a resource

Human wastes are regarded as a resource in many parts of the world, and they are widely used for a large variety of purposes (see Table 2.1). These Guidelines emphasize the following three reuse practices, since these are the most common:

- wastewater use in agriculture (crop irrigation);

- excreta use in agriculture (soil fertilization); and

- wastewater and excreta use in aquaculture (fish culture, aquatic macrophyte production).

2.1 Wastewater use in agriculture

With the introduction of the water-carriage system for domestic wastewater in the middle of the nineteenth century, many European and North American cities adopted crop irrigation as their means of wastewater disposal. Sewage farms, as they were called, were established in the United Kingdom as early as 1865, the United States in 1871, France in 1872, Germany in 1876, India in 1877, Australia in 1893 and Mexico in 1904. In most of these countries the impetus for sewage farming was to prevent river pollution rather than to enhance crop production; in the United Kingdom the dictum was "sewage to the land, rain to the rivers". However, as cities grew and the proportion of their population connected to sewer systems increased, the land area required for sewage farming became too great. The practice became less popular and, with the development of modern wastewater treatment processes such as biofiltration and activated sludge during the first two decades of this century, it disappeared completely in many countries soon after the First World War, since wastewaters could be readily discharged to surface waters without causing significant pollution. The sewage farms at Werribee (Melbourne, Australia) and Mexico City were notable exceptions to this trend, and they are still in operation some 80–90 years after their

Table 2.1 Examples of human wastes reuse practices

Reuse practice	Responsible social unit	Examples
Soil fertilization with untreated stored nightsoil	Family or community	China, India, Japan, Thailand
Nightsoil collected and composted for use in agriculture	Community or local authority	China, India
Nightsoil fed to animals	Family	Africa, Melanesia
Use of compost latrines	Family	Guatemala, United Republic of Tanzania, Viet Nam
Biogas production	Family or community	China, India
Fish pond fertilization with treated or untreated nightsoil	Family or community	China, Indonesia, Malaysia
Fish farming in stabilization ponds	Family (illegal) or commercial farmer	India, Israel, Kenya
Aquatic weed production in ponds	Family, community or local authority	S.E. Asia, Viet Nam
Agricultural application of wastewater	Local authority or commercial farmer	See Table 2.2
Agricultural application of wastewater sludges	Local authority or commercial farmer	Kenya, United Kingdom, United States of America
Irrigation with stabilization pond effluents	Local authority or commercial farmer	India, Israel, Peru
Algal production in stabilization ponds	Local authority	Israel, Japan, Mexico

Source: Strauss (1985)

inception. However, indirect reuse — the use of water from rivers receiving wastewater effluents — occurs throughout the world, and is currently the most common process of using effluents not only for irrigation but also, after appropriate treatment, for potable supplies.

In the past two decades there has been a great increase in the use of wastewater for crop irrigation (see Table 2.2), especially in semiarid

Table 2.2 Global data on wastewater irrigation

Country and city	Irrigated area (ha)
Argentina, Mendoza	3 700
Australia, Melbourne	10 000
Bahrain, Tubli	800
Chile, Santiago	16 000
China, all cities	1 330 000
Federal Republic of Germany, Braunschweig	3 000
Other cities	25 000
India, Calcutta	12 500
All cities	73 000
Israel, several cities	8 800
Kuwait, several cities[a]	12 000
Mexico, Mexico City	90 000
All cities[a]	250 000
Peru, Lima[a]	6 800
Saudi Arabia, Riyadh	2 850
South Africa, Johannesburg	1 800
Sudan, Khartoum	2 800
Tunisia, Tunis[a]	4 450
Other cities[a]	2 900
United States of America, Chandler, Arizona	2 800
Bakersfield, California	2 250
Fresno, California	1 625
Santa Rosa, California	1 600
Lubbock, Texas	3 000
Muskegon, Michigan	2 200

[a] Includes planned expansion of existing reuse

Source: Bartone & Arlosoroff (1987)

areas of both developed and developing countries (see Figure 2.1). This has occurred as a result of several factors:

- the scarcity of alternative waters for irrigation;

- the high cost of artificial fertilizers;

- the demonstration that health risks and soil damage are minimal if the necessary precautions are taken;

- the high cost of advanced wastewater treatment plants;

- the sociocultural acceptance of the practice; and

Figure 2.1 Irrigation with treated wastewater in Saudi Arabia
The irrigated fields are in stark contrast to the natural arid terrain.

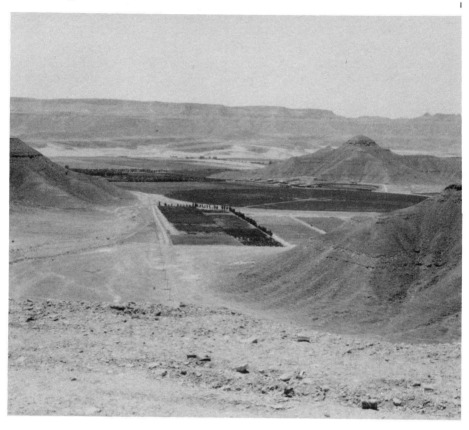

- the recognition by water resource planners of the value of the practice.

Domestic wastewater is produced by households that have an in-house multiple-tap water supply service and flush-toilets connected to a sewer system into which all other household wastewater (sullage) is discharged. In the developing world as a whole, few households produce sewage, because sewerage is too expensive a sanitation technology; the majority produce excreta (nightsoil) and sullage separately. In many urban areas, however, sufficient households are connected to a sewer system to make the agricultural use of sewage an attractive economic proposition: crops are both irrigated and fertilized by the water and nutrients in sewage. At the same time the wasteful disposal of these scarce resources, which often leads to gross environmental pollution, is avoided. With proper management, crop

Box 2.1 Wastewater irrigation increases crop yields

There are many reports from all over the world that crop yields are significantly increased by irrigation with wastewater. In India, for example, long-term field experiments at the National Environmental Engineering Research Institute in Nagpur have shown that medium intensity irrigation with wastewater produces higher yields than irrigation with freshwater supplemented with standard doses of nitrogen, phosphorus and potassium (NPK), as shown in the table below.

	Crop yields (tonnes per hectare per year)				
Irrigation water	**Wheat**	**Moong beans**	**Rice**	**Potato**	**Cotton**
	(8)[a]	**(5)**	**(7)**	**(4)**	**(3)**
Raw wastewater	3.34	0.90	2.97	23.11	2.56
Settled wastewater	3.45	0.87	2.94	20.78	2.30
Stabilization pond effluent	3.45	0.78	2.98	22.31	2.41
Fresh water + NPK	2.70	0.72	2.03	17.16	1.70

[a] Years of harvest used to calculate average yield

Source: Shende (1985).

yields are increased (see Box 2.1) and no adverse health effects are induced. In current practice wastewater irrigation of crops sometimes does lead to an excess of excreta-related disease among farm labourers and crop consumers, but this is entirely due to the use of inappropriate techniques. It is now possible to design and implement wastewater use schemes that avoid the transmission of excreta-related infections, and thus potential health risks, which are now wholly avoidable (see Section 4), should no longer be considered sufficient reason not to continue and develop this otherwise very beneficial practice.

Some governments have been understandably cautious in actively promoting wastewater use, especially as there has not, until recently, been either a realistic appraisal of the health risks involved, or sensible design guidelines for treatment of wastewater before use. However, no such caution is shown in practice by those who actually use the wastewater — farmers and market gardeners — and throughout the developing world untreated wastewater is commonly used to irrigate agricultural and horticultural produce. Indeed, in many areas wastewater is considered to be so valuable that sewers are broken into and the wastewater flow is diverted to the fields. Such a practice, which is by no means uncommon but of course is illegal and carries substantial health risks, clearly demonstrates the perceived advantage of wastewater use. It is doubtful whether such practices can ever be eliminated unless governments develop and promulgate national strategies for wastewater use. Proper measures to minimize health risks and ensure the equitable distribution of the wastewater for irrigation are the only means by which the potential economic advantage of wastewater use can be maximized, and its actual health risks eliminated.

Water

Wastewater is composed of 99.9% water and 0.1% other material (suspended, colloidal and dissolved solids). In arid and semi-arid areas water resources are so scarce that there is often a major conflict between urban (domestic and industrial) and agricultural demands for water. This conflict can usually be resolved only by the agricultural use of wastewater: the cities must use the fresh water first, and urban wastewater — after proper treatment (see Section 7) — is then used for crop irrigation. If such a sequence of water resource utilization is not followed, both urban and agricultural development may be seriously constrained, with consequent adverse effects on national economic development.

The rate of wastewater generation is usually between 80 and 200 litres per person per day, or some 30–70 m³ per person per year. Thus in semi-arid areas with a water demand of, for example, 2 m per year (the range is commonly 1.5–3 m per year), one person's wastewater could be used to irrigate 15–35 m² of land. In other words, a city of one million people will produce enough wastewater to irrigate approximately 1500–3500 ha.

Nutrients

The suspended, colloidal and dissolved solids present in wastewater contain major plant nutrients (nitrogen, phosphorus and potassium) and also trace nutrients (such as copper, iron and zinc). Total nitrogen and phosphorus concentrations in raw wastewater are usually in the ranges 10–100 mg/litre and 5–25 mg/litre respectively, and potassium is in the range 10–40 mg/litre. Treated wastewaters will contain less nitrogen and phosphorus, but approximately the same amount of potassium, depending on the treatment process used. For the irrigation rate of 2 m per year commonly required in semi-arid climates, concentrations of 15 and 3 mg/litre of total nitrogen and total phosphorus respectively in well treated domestic wastewater (such as can be expected in the final effluent of a well designed series of waste stabilization ponds) correspond to annual nitrogen and phosphorus application rates of 300 and 60 kg/ha respectively. Supplementary fertilizer requirements can thus be reduced, or even eliminated, by wastewater irrigation.

Contaminants and toxins

In addition to beneficial nutrients wastewater also contains contaminants and toxins. The contaminants are the excreted pathogens — disease-causing viruses, bacteria, protozoa and helminths — which are present in variable numbers in all wastewaters. In Europe, for example, domestic wastewater often contains some 10^4 salmonella bacteria per litre; in developing countries pathogen numbers and diversity are much greater. The health risks posed by these pathogens are discussed in Section 4, and treatment processes for removing pathogens before irrigation are described in Section 7.

Wastewater, especially if it includes a significant proportion of industrial effluent, may contain compounds that are toxic to both humans and plants. Heavy metals are an obvious example, but boron (derived from synthetic detergents) is an important phytotoxin, especially of citrus crops. Provided that the quality of the wastewater conforms to that recommended by the Food and Agriculture Organization of the United Nations for irrigation water (Ayers & Westcot, 1984), it may be safely used for crop irrigation. Domestic and normal municipal wastewaters are usually of adequate physicochemical quality for crop irrigation, and only the boron sensitivity of the irrigated crop requires particular attention.

Application rate

The application rate of wastewater to crops is calculated in the same way as for irrigation with fresh water, with due regard to evapotranspiration demand, leaching requirements and salinity and sodicity control (Pettygrove & Asano, 1984).

2.2 Excreta use in agriculture

The application of excreta to the land to fertilize crops (Figure 2.2) is a common practice in China and Viet Nam, for example, and in the

Figure 2.2 Application of nightsoil to crops in China (Province of Taiwan)

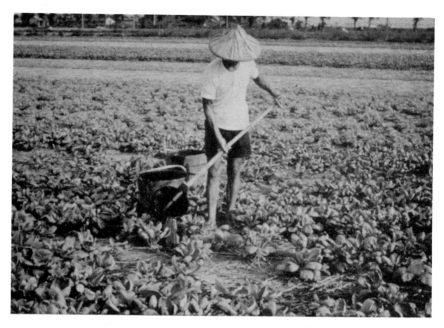

recent past this was also true in Japan. It is the only agricultural use option in areas without a sewerage system and, since the majority of households lack such systems (a condition that is likely to persist for at least the foreseeable future), excreta use has greater agricultural potential than wastewater use. Emphasis should thus be directed towards the implementation of on-site sanitation technologies that readily permit the use of stored excreta — for example, alternating twin-pit or pour-flush latrines and compost toilets as used in such places as Guatemala and Viet Nam.

Historically the importance of excreta use in agriculture may be judged by the experience in China, where soil fertility has been maintained by this practice for thousands of years (see Box 2.2). In 1965, for example, approximately 90% of all human excreta produced in China was used as fertilizer, and this amounted to 22% of all plant nutrients used, including those derived from chemical fertilizers; a further 25% was derived from the use of animal manure (Chao, 1970). In addition to supplying nutrients, excreta are very valuable in increasing the humus content of the soil, which significantly improves the structure and water-retaining capacity of the soil. Notwithstanding the clear agricultural and horticultural advantages, there is in many societies a strong sociocultural aversion to the

---

Box 2.2 Agricultural utilization of excreta in Eastern Asia

One of the most remarkable agricultural practices adopted by any civilised people is the centuries-long and well-nigh universal conservation of all human waste in China, Korea and Japan .... The human manure saved and applied to the fields of Japan in 1908 amounted to 23 850 295 tons [21 636 988 tonnes], which is an average of 1.75 tons per acre [3.92 t/ha] of their 21 321 square miles [55 226 km²] of cultivated land in the four main islands .... In Eastern Asia for more than thirty centuries, these wastes have been religiously saved, and today the 400 millions of adult population send back to their fields annually 150 000 tons [136 000 t] of phosphorus, 376 000 tons [341 000 t] of potassium and 1 158 000 tons [1 051 000 t] of nitrogen comprised in a gross weight exceeding 182 000 000 tons [165 000 000 t].

Source: King (1926)

---

agricultural and horticultural use of excreta (see Section 5), although the use of some excreta-derived products is common and socially acceptable. In the United Kingdom, for example, 47% of all wastewater sludge is applied to land (Water Authorities Association, 1985).

The agricultural and horticultural use of excreta has the potential to promote the transmission of excreta-related disease, especially if raw excreta are applied to the land. However, as in the case of wastewater use, it is now possible to design and operate excreta use schemes in which pathogen transfer via excreta-fertilized crops, even including salad crops eaten raw, is eliminated (see Section 7). It is thus no longer necessary to consider excreta use as a practice that automatically causes disease transmission, and attention can be shifted to its clear agricultural and horticultural advantages.

Excreta quality

Because of differences in diet and climatic factors, there is considerable variation in the quantity of excreta produced, but a typical value for urban areas of developing countries is 1.8 litres per person per day (Feachem et al., 1983). In this volume there are approximately 350 grams of dry solids which comprise around 90 grams of organic

Table 2.3 Approximate nutrient content of various natural fertilizers

Type of fertilizer	Nutrient content (% of dry weight)		
	Total N	P_2O_5	K_2O
Human faeces	5–7	3–5.4	1–2.5
Human urine	15–19	2.5–5	3–4.5
Fresh nightsoil[a]	10.4–13.1	2.7–5.1	2.1–3.5
Fresh cattle manure	0.3–1.9	0.1–0.7	0.3–1.2
Pig manure	4–6	3–4	2.5–3
Plant residues	1–11	0.5–2.8	1.1–11

[a] Faeces, urine and 0.35 litres of ablution water

Source: Strauss (1985)

matter and significant quantities of plant nutrients (see Table 2.3). Treatment of excreta, in addition to destroying pathogens, improves quality principally by stabilizing the organic matter so that it is a better soil conditioner and by converting the nutrients to forms more readily used by plants. The physicochemical and microbiological qualities of excreta-derived materials (for example sludge from latrines and septic tanks, composted nightsoil and wastewater sludges) depend on the degree of treatment given, and should be regularly monitored before application to crops.

Application rates

Excreta and excreta-derived materials are often applied to the land before crop planting, at an annual rate of approximately 5–30 t/ha depending on the available concentrations of nutrients and the crops being fertilized. These are not high rates of application—10 t/ha, for example, is equal to only 1 kg/m² —and supplementary fertilization may be required to obtain maximal yields.

Urban nightsoil, if it contains small quantities of toilet flushwater in addition to excreta (such that its volume is some 5–10 litres per person per day), is often used, especially in Eastern Asia, for crop irrigation as well as fertilization. In such cases the application rate depends on the consumption demands of the crop, although supplementary irrigation may be advisable to prevent wastage of the nutrients present in the nightsoil.

2.3 Excreta and wastewater use in aquaculture

Aquaculture means "water-farming", just as agriculture means "field-farming", and it refers to the ancient practices of fish culture, notably of carp and tilapia, and the growing of certain aquatic crops, such as water spinach (*Ipomoea aquatica*), water chestnut (*Eleocharis dulcis* and *E. tuberosa*), water hyacinth (*Eichhornia crassipes*), water calthrop (*Trapa* spp) and lotus (*Nelumbo nucifera*). The fertilization of aquaculture ponds with human wastes has been practised for thousands of years in Asia (Figure 2.3), and today at least two-thirds of the world yield of farmed fish is obtained from ponds fertilized with excreta and animal manure. Such fish represent the cheapest source of animal protein. The Chinese experience, especially their integration of aquaculture with agriculture (see Box 2.3), is an

---

Box 2.3 Integration of aquaculture and agriculture in China

"Aquaculture in China is a part of the overall agricultural farming system. It is either carried out as a primary farm occupation, or as a secondary or sideline activity depending on the extent and nature of land and water resources available. This integration of farming activities provides a vivid demonstration of how the full use of all raw materials available in the farm can be cycled into the production of food. Animal manures are used to fertilize the ponds and croplands; the land, in turn, produces food crops for animals, fish and man; the wastes of fish accumulated in the pond are recycled back to the soil where land crops are grown. This illustrates the practical reasons for integration and diversification of land and water farming.

"Integration of aquaculture with agriculture is carried out on only a limited scale in other countries, unlike the full integration that is found in China. A major reason for this is the difference in the control of the means of production, and in the ownership of resources used for production. Most countries have private land ownership systems where it is difficult to implement a unified development strategy. In China, land is state-owned and development programmes are centrally directed even though implementation is highly decentralized. This gives flexibility at the local level in undertaking their respective production activities, but at the same time maintains central control over the resources decisive for nationwide development. Local needs and experience are the basis of planning, which provides a strong motivation for rural production and development."

Source: Tapiador et al. (1977)

Figure 2.3 Application of nightsoil to fishponds in China

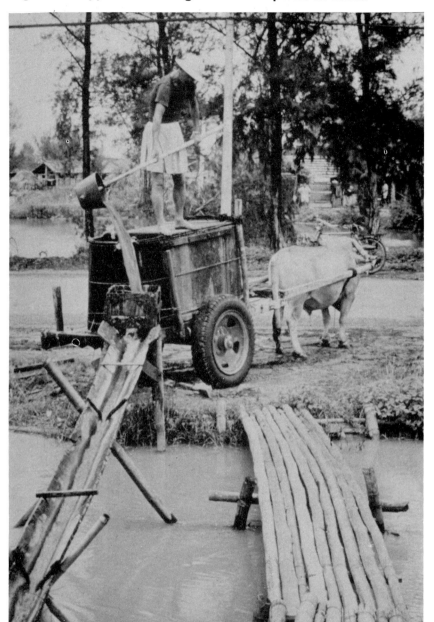

important example of waste-based aquaculture. China produces 60% of the world's farmed fish in only 27% of the world's area of fish-ponds (2.25 million tonnes per year from 7000 km² of ponds in China, compared with 1.5 million tonnes per year from 18 000 km² of ponds in the rest of the world). The mean yield in Chinese fish-ponds is 3200 kilograms per hectare per year, but in well managed intensive polyculture ponds the yield can be up to 7000 kilograms per hectare per year (Wohlfarth, 1978).

The use of untreated excreta to fertilize fish is becoming less common in many parts of the world, and in China excreta are now used only after storage for four weeks in closed containers (Tapiador et al., 1977). In addition to excreta, wastewater sludge, biogas slurry, septage and excreta-derived compost can all be used to fertilize fish-ponds (Polprasert et al., 1982; Huggins, 1985; Zandstra, 1986). More recent aquacultural developments have been the culture and harvesting of microalgae in high-rate algal ponds, and the raising of valuable crustaceans such as shrimps and crayfish.

Fish can be successfully raised in the maturation ponds of a series of waste stabilization ponds (Bartone, 1985; Payne, 1985), and annual yields of up to 3000 kilograms per hectare have been obtained. Care is needed to maintain aerobic conditions and to keep unionized ammonia levels low (<0.5 mg nitrogen/litre) in order to avoid fish kills (Bartone et al., 1985). The sale of harvested fish can be used to pay for improved operation and maintenance of municipal sewerage systems in developing countries (Meadows, 1983).

Application rates

Despite the very large number of reports describing the successful culture of fish and aquatic macrophytes in ponds fertilized with excreta and wastewater, there are almost no data on excreta and wastewater application rates. The fish-ponds at Munich, Federal Republic of Germany, which are fertilized with settled wastewater, receive an annual mean organic loading in the range 33–77 kilograms BOD (biochemical oxygen demand) per hectare per day (Edwards, 1985). On the basis of a design loading of 50 kilograms BOD per hectare per day and a per caput BOD contribution of 25 grams per day (for settled wastewater or raw nightsoil), this corresponds to 1 hectare of fish-pond for every 2000 people. In China, however, excreta and animal manures are applied to fish-ponds at an annual rate of up to 40 000 kg/ha, corresponding to approximately 1 hectare of pond for every 45 pigs or 115 people (Tapiador et al., 1977). Advice for small-scale fish farming operations is given by Edwards & Kaewpaitoon (1984), but clearly further work is needed to develop more rational guidelines for loading fish-ponds with human wastes.

3
Examples of human wastes reuse

Wastewater irrigation schemes in Australia, the Federal Republic of Germany, India, Mexico and Tunisia are described in this section, as is the use of excreta or excreta-derived products in China, Guatemala, India and the United States of America. Descriptions of the aquacultural use of wastewater and excreta for fish culture in India and Indonesia are also given. There are many other examples of waste reuse (see Table 2.1, page 24); the selection given here was chosen to represent a wide range of geographical locations, sociocultural settings, scales of operation, treatment processes, application techniques and crops harvested.

3.1 Wastewater use in agriculture

3.1.1 Australia

Werribee Farm came into service as the principal sewage farm for the city of Melbourne in 1897, when the design population was 1 million. Today Werribee Farm receives an average flow of some 470 000 m³/day of mixed domestic and industrial wastewater. This is treated either in waste stabilization ponds (1500 ha in area), or by land or grass filtration. Land filtration covers an area of nearly 4000 ha and treats a wastewater flow of some 195 000 m³/day during the summer months of October–April. It is essentially the broad irrigation of pasture with raw wastewater. Irrigation is carried out on a three-weekly rotational basis: two days of wastewater application totalling 100 mm, followed by five days drying and then 2 weeks of grazing by livestock, mainly sheep and cattle. Some 10–11 applications of wastewater are made each season. Approximately half the wastewater is lost by evapotranspiration and seepage into the deep subsoil, and the remainder is collected by a series of effluent drains and eventually discharged into Port Philip Bay (Kirby, 1967). As a wastewater treatment process, it is very efficient: biochemical oxygen demand and suspended solids removal of 98% and 93% are achieved. During winter, land filtration is not feasible because of the lower rates of evapotranspiration, and grass filtration is practised instead. A flow of some 250 000 m³/day of primary settled sewage is treated in an area of 1500 ha. At the end of the season cattle are admitted to feed on the pasture following seed-drop.

The farm carries a large number of livestock. There is a herd of some 13 000 adult cattle, which produce around 6500 calves each winter; most of these calves are fattened and sold at 18–22 months old. Only 0.02% of carcasses are condemned for contamination with *Cysticercus bovis* (beef tapeworm larva), which is a similar rate to that for cattle from other local farms; this demonstrates the effectiveness of the irrigation regime in preventing tapeworm transmission. In summer the farm has about 30 000 sheep; most of these are sold in the autumn, except for 6000 which are retained for winter grazing. These stockraising activities generate a gross annual income of some A\$3 million (US\$ 2.12 million) (Camp Scott Furphy Pty Ltd, 1986).

3.1.2 Federal Republic of Germany

Crop irrigation with treated wastewater has been practised at the city of Brunswick (Braunschweig; current population 325 000) in northern Federal Republic of Germany since 1971 (Kayser, 1985). Some 55 000 m³/day of wastewater are treated in aerated lagoons and secondary sedimentation tanks, and 44 500 m³/day (which includes 5100 m³/day unthickened excess sludge and 5000 m³/day raw wastewater from villages near the irrigation fields) are used to irrigate 2800 ha of farmland. The irrigation scheme is operated and managed by the Brunswick Wastewater Utilization Association (BWUA), whose members are the city of Brunswick and the 440 individual farmers who own the land. The irrigation area is divided into four irrigation districts, each with its own pumping station and wastewater balancing tank. The wastewater is distributed by subsurface asbestos cement pressure pipes (100–500 mm diameter), and subsurface hydrants are located 90 m apart. Wastewater is applied to the crops by means of sprinklers (20 mm nozzle diameter) attached to drum-coiled irrigation machines. During normal operation the sprinkler takes 20 hours to apply 50 mm of wastewater at a pressure of 4 bars (400 kPa) to a strip of land measuring 300 m × 50 m. Usually 50–60 machines are in operation, although this may rise to 100 in summer when ground water is also used for irrigation;

six heavy-duty tractors are used to position the machines and pull out the 300 m sprinkler pipe over the field. Each tractor is manned by a crew of two in summer and one in winter when low pressure irrigation is practised essentially as a wastewater disposal technique.

The annual wastewater application rate is 580 mm, and the applied nutrient loads (kg/ha per year) are: nitrogen 379, phosphorus 106 and potassium 105. The light, very permeable soil requires liming to maintain the pH, and supplementary potassium and nitrogen fertilizers are used. The principal crops grown are winter and summer grain, sugar-beet and potatoes. Yields are similar to those from fields irrigated with ground water and artificially fertilized.

Only a small fraction of the total wastewater applied to the fields is collected in tile drains and discharged to a local river; most is either evaporated or flows into the ground water. Final effluent quality is high (<1 mg BOD per litre), although the nitrate concentration of 25 mg nitrogen/litre is giving rise to serious concern. No problems have been encountered with heavy metal accumulation in the soil.

Health risks are minimized by prohibiting the growth of vegetables and fruits in the irrigation area, and by a BWUA irrigation decree to eliminate the spread of pathogens from the sprinklers. This decree stipulates that 10-m wide hedges have to be planted along borders with public roads and that irrigation should not take place within 50 m of public roads and 100 m of houses. Special low-level sprinklers have to be used within 115 m of roads and houses, and sprinkler operation closer than 100 m to roads is permitted only when the wind direction is from the road to the field. Irrigation is ceased three weeks before crops are harvested. Investigations have indicated that these measures are sufficient to control disease transmission.

The BWUA irrigation scheme is strictly managed. An irrigation schedule is worked out every year in winter according to the farmers' cultivation plans. In summer, depending on the actual weather conditions, the schedule is refined each week. BWUA staff are responsible for operating the whole irrigation system, maintaining the pumping stations, moving the irrigation machines and for general maintenance and repair. In addition two employees act as internal controllers to ensure that the irrigation decree is rigidly observed.

Energy consumption is high, approximately 0.5 kWh per cubic metre of wastewater treated and irrigated, or some 8 million kWh per year. Operating costs are correspondingly high, amounting to nearly DM 8 million (US$ 4 million) per year, of which the farmers pay 5% at a rate of DM 120 (US$ 60) per hectare of irrigated land. The city of Brunswick pays the remainder, and justifies this cost on the basis that the scheme serves as an effective sludge disposal system, as well as an advanced tertiary wastewater treatment system.

3.1.3 India

A recent report prepared for the Food and Agriculture Organization of the United Nations (Shende, 1985) indicates that there are over 200 wastewater irrigation schemes currently in operation in India, covering an area of approximately 73 000 ha. Many of these schemes, however, are operated "in a crude and irrational manner" and with substantial actual health risks since most of the wastewater used for irrigation is untreated (see Section 4.3). Excessive wastewater application rates are used (up to 12 m per year), resulting in very high nutrient loading rates (up to 600 kg total nitrogen per hectare per year), because most schemes are operated more for wastewater disposal than for optimal resource recovery. Information on 13 major schemes is given in Table 3.1. Irrigation is by surface application methods, ranging from uncontrolled flooding to fairly well managed ridge and furrow, border strip and check basin irrigation. Subsurface and sprinkler irrigation are not practised on sewage farms in India.

Despite this generally discouraging picture of the current status of wastewater irrigation in India, there are some noteworthy successes. Experience gained by the National Environmental Engineering Research Institute (NEERI) from long-term field studies indicates that:

- Grain yields are significantly improved by wastewater irrigation compared with irrigation with fresh water alone, even when raw wastewater is diluted with two volumes of fresh water. Yields can be increased further by adding supplementary NPK fertilizer up to the recommended dose.

- Vegetable yields are also much higher when wastewater irrigation is practised instead of traditional manuring and freshwater irrigation (see Table 3.2).

39

Table 3.1 Details of thirteen sewage farms in India

Location	Area (ha)	Volume of sewage used (mld)[a]	Treatment, if any	Dilution if any	Application rates (m³/day/ha)	Soil type	Crops grown
Ahmedabad	890.3	299.9	Nil	Nil	336.8	Sandy loam	Pochia grass, paddy, maize, jowar, wheat, lucerne
Amritsar	1214.1	54.5	Nil	1:3	44.9	Sandy clay	Maize, berseem, sorghum, lucerne
Bikaner	40.4	13.6	Nil	Nil	336.8	Sandy	Bajra, wheat, grasses, vegetables
Bhilai	607	36.3	Secondary (stablization pond)	Nil	59.9	Sandy loam, clay loam	Paddy, maize, wheat, tuwar, vegetables
Delhi	1214.1	227.2	Primary and secondary	Nil	187.1	Sandy loam, loamy sand	Jowar, bajra, maize, barley, wheat, pulses, vegetables
Gwalior	202.3	11.3	Nil	Nil	56.1	Silt loam, clay loam	Paddy, maize andguar, jowar, cowpea, wheat, potato, berseem, vegetables
Hyderabad	607	95.4	Primary	1:1.5	157.2	Loam	Para-grass, paddy
Jamshedpur	113.3	9.1	Secondary acti-vated sludge	Nil	80.2	Clay loam	Napier grass, para-grass, guinea grass, berseem, jowar, maize
Kanpur	1416.5	31.8	Nil	1:1	22.4	Loam, silt loam	Wheat, paddy, maize, barley, potato, oats, vegetablLs
Madras	133.5	6.8	Nil	Nil	51.0	Sandy to silt loam	Para-grass.
Madurai	76.9	136	Nil	Nil	177.3	Red sandy loam	Guinea grass
Trivandrum	37.2	8.6	Nil	1:1	231.9	Sand	Para-grass
Lucknow	150	300	Nil	1:3	–	Sandy loam	Maize, paddy, potato, vegetables, fruits, papaya, plantains, citrus

[a] Million litres per day
Reproduced by permission from Shende (1985).

Table 3.2 Yields of crops irrigated with canal water and diluted and undiluted wastewater at Poona sewage farm

Crop	Annual crop yield (t/ha)		
	Canal water[a]	Diluted wastewater[b]	Undiluted wastewater
Beetroot	8.75	15.60	16.27
Carrot	9.71	8.72	11.75
Radish	7.26	6.14	8.33
Turmeric	–	20.64	21.59
Potato	6.12	7.00	9.33
Ginger	6.04	9.18	9.80
Papaya	26.72	27.91	37.00
Kholkhol	9.70	11.76	16.57
Cabbage	9.27	11.32	12.13
Cauliflower	6.96	7.08	9.09
Okra	2.82	3.60	5.89
French beans	6.63	8.20	8.06
Tomato	10.01	–	13.38
Tobacco	1.12	1.25	1.25
Groundnut	2.88	2.90	3.17
Sugar (cane)	–	52.75	54.43
Sugar (jaggery)	–	5.67	5.78

[a] Land manured before planting
[b] 1 : 1 dilution

Reproduced by permission from Shende (1985).

- Irrigation with wastewater results in a higher nutrient utilization efficiency, and permits higher yields to be maintained in the long term (see Box 2.1, page 27).

- Irrigation of trees with raw wastewater results in yields similar to those obtained from freshwater irrigation — approximately 55 tonnes of marketable eucalyptus timber per hectare after 24 months, with a market value of Rs 27 700 (US$ 2170).

- The effect of wastewater irrigation on soil properties depends strongly on the original soil characteristics, but in many cases — even after 30 years of wastewater irrigation — soil productivity remains highly favourable.

3.1.4 Mexico

Agricultural development in Mexico is highly dependent on irrigation: 77% of the land is arid or semi-arid and the mean annual rainfall for the whole country is only 760 mm, occurring mainly between July and September. Wastewater use in agriculture is practised throughout the country in almost every city that has a sewerage system. In some irrigation districts a blend of wastewater and fresh water is used, but in Rural Development District No. 063 in the Mezquital Valley, State of Hidalgo, almost all the water used for irrigation is the wastewater from Mexico City and its metropolitan area, which has a total population of 18 million. The wastewater is used for crop irrigation in two Irrigation Districts (Nos 03 and 100); these comprise a total of 85 000 ha of irrigable land, of which 80 000 ha are currently irrigated. The principal crops grown are alfalfa, maize, wheat, oats, beans, tomatoes, chillies and beetroot. The combined wastewater and storm water flow of 55 m³/s, of which 30–45 m³/s is raw wastewater, makes the Mexico City wastewater use scheme the largest in the world (Villalobos et al., 1981; Duron, 1985; Strauss, 1986a; Romero-Alvarez, personal communication, 1987).

The combined wastewater and storm water from Mexico City flows in three large canals to the Tula basin which lies to the north of the city. This area, which is some 2000 m above sea level and has an average temperature of 17 °C, is semi-arid: annual rainfall averages 483 mm and evaporation 810 mm. Irrigation is thus essential for successful agriculture. No treatment *per se* is given to the wastewater, but a certain degree of treatment occurs naturally during its 60 km journey from Mexico City to Tula. Further treatment takes place in storage reservoirs which are used to regulate the flow to the irrigation canals. Some of these storage reservoirs also impound local rivers, thus diluting the wastewater.

In Irrigation District No. 03, within the Tula basin, there are approximately 200 km of main irrigation canals and 350 km of lateral channels covering an area of 43 000 ha. Irrigation water usage, much of which is regulated by several reservoirs, amounts to 1–1.4 × 10⁹ m³ per year. Data on irrigation water quality are scanty, but there have been no serious problems with salinity, sodicity or heavy metals over the past 30 years, despite the generally low quality of the irrigation water. This is attributed to the good internal drainage and high calcium content of the local soils which have prevented the accumulation of dissolved salts and exchangeable sodium. The crops grown are tolerant to the relatively high levels of boron present in the irrigation waters, but some crops irrigated with wastewater (for example alfalfa) have shown higher concentrations of heavy metals (cadmium, chromium, selenium and zinc) than those irrigated with fresh water. No detailed information on bacteriological quality is available, but some samples have contained between 10^3 and 10^8 faecal coliforms per 100 ml.

The Irrigation District produces a considerable quantity of food, mainly for the markets of Mexico City and local consumption (see Figure 3.1). In addition to the main crops shown in Table 3.3, vegetables are grown on some 400 ha; there is enforced crop restriction, and those that cannot be grown include lettuce, cabbage, beetroot, coriander, radish, carrot, spinach and parsley. The District's canal and gate operators, who are in close contact with the farmers, are responsible for ensuring that these crops are not grown. There is also a small, but valuable, production of fruit and flowers. Research into oil-bearing crops (sunflower, safflower and rape) is in progress.

Administratively the Irrigation Districts, which were established in their present form by presidential decree in 1955, are controlled by a committee composed of representatives of central government (the Secretariat of Agriculture and Water Resources, SARH), the farmers and local credit banks. The responsibilities of the District comprise:

- construction, operation and maintenance of the irrigation and drainage canals;

- maintenance of access roads;

- allocation of irrigation water to farmers;

- administration of farmers' crop-growing schedules;

- enforcement of prohibited crop ordinances; and

- provision of an agricultural extension service to the farmers.

The Irrigation Districts Nos. 03 and 100 are divided into several administrative areas. Farmers place their water demands with their local District office, specifying where and when the water is required. The farmers, who are either individual

Figure 3.1 A farm in Mexico's Irrigation District 03, irrigated with untreated wastewater from Mexico City

The small boy is not wearing shoes, and is therefore exposed to hookworm infection because of the flood irrigation method in use

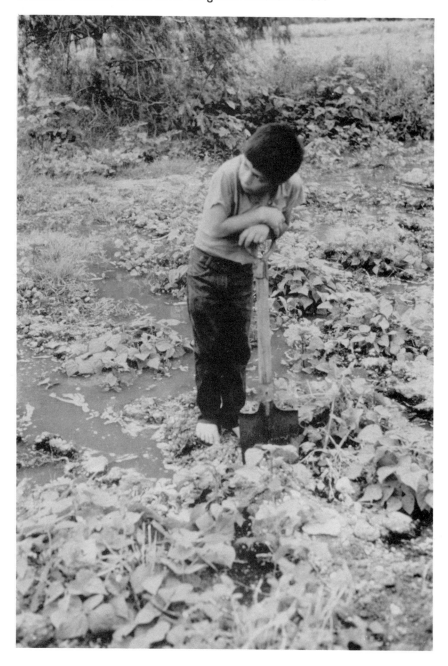

Table 3.3 Yields of principal crops and areas harvested in Irrigation District No. 03, Mezquital Valley, Mexico

Crop		Area harvested (ha) and yield (kg/ha)			
		1970–71	1975–76	1980–81	1985–86
Maize	Harvested (ha)	17 914	21 023	17 907	19 539
	Yield (kg/ha)	3 938	3 896	4 566	4 600
Beans	Harvested (ha)	1 266	1 222	1 646	1 501
	Yield (kg/ha)	1 259	1 768	1 521	1 800
Wheat	Harvested (ha)	7 293	2 634	2 005	167
	Yield (kg/ha)	1 919	3 119	3 225	2 900
Alfalfa	Harvested (ha)	12 708	15 206	20 339	20 630
	Yield (kg/ha)	95 300	89 154	91 175	81 200
Oats	Harvested (ha)	2 998	691	1 002	1 592
	Yield (kg/ha)	18 150	19 898	32 470	23 600
Barley	Harvested (ha)	–	832	1 812	1 514
	Yield (kg/ha)	–	19 620	19 939	15 500
Pastures	Harvested (ha)	13	11	65	30
	Yield (kg/ha)	142 500	107 000	44 276	89 100

Source: Duron (1985) and Secretariat of Agriculture and Water Resources (personal communication).

smallholders or work in cooperatives, pay a water fee of 40 pesos (US$ 0.12) per hectare per irrigation cycle (approximately 20 pesos (US$ 0.06) per 1000 m³), which is insufficient to permit full cost recovery—subsidies are received from the State. Farmers irrigate every 25–30 days.

The success of the Mexico City wastewater use scheme has been dependent upon a number of factors, including:

- the suitability of the local soils for wastewater irrigation;

- the highly increased soil productivity resulting from wastewater irrigation, which makes it possible to grow more than one crop per year;

- the availability of large tracts of originally semi-arid land;

- a highly developed and well maintained wastewater distribution system;

- enhanced security for the local farmers, who do not have to rely on rain-fed agriculture but have the use of steadily increasing amounts of wastewater;

- sound management of the wastewater irrigation districts, which have over 80 years of experience of wastewater irrigation; and

- the absence of any demonstrated risk of the transmission of excreta-related disease.

3.1.5 Tunisia

Tunisia is a highly agricultural country; of its total land area of 160 000 km², some 90 000 km² are cultivated, and 50% of the country's 7 million people live in rural areas. The main products are wheat, barley, citrus fruits, olives, dates and wine, and the value of agricultural exports is high. Little rainfall occurs in the summer, and irrigated agriculture is well developed. Wastewater use is becoming increasingly common, as alternative water sources (impoundments, ground water) become insufficient in quantity and quality. To avoid over-pumping ground water, a major use has been found for wastewater in preventing the intrusion of salt water into coastal aquifers. Currently there are twelve reuse schemes, with three more being implemented and plans for a further five (Strauss, 1986b). Most of the wastewater used for irrigation is secondary effluent but some sewage treatment plant sludge is also being utilized. A wide variety of crops is cultivated — citrus and other fruit trees (Figure 3.2), fodder crops, and vegetables. In one tourist location, a golf course is watered with activated sludge effluent.

Wastewater from the capital city of Tunis has been reused for the irrigation of citrus trees since 1964. Some 600 ha of land are irrigated in the neighbouring district of Soukra, and there are new schemes under implementation that will expand wastewater use to about 5000 ha in three principal irrigation districts around Tunis in the near future. The effluents from four treatment plants (two activated sludge, one waste stabilization pond complex and one oxidation ditch), totalling some 250 000 m³/day, will be used. The waste stabilization ponds, at Côtière Nord, comprise two parallel series of three ponds (the first of which is mechanically aerated) which discharge into a common quaternary pond. The overall retention time is currently 180 days, and, at the maximum design flow, 58 days; the bacteriological quality of the effluent is certainly well

Figure 3.2 A citrus orchard in Tunisia, irrigated with treated wastewater
Buried pipes distribute the water and riser ("bubbler") pipes apply it to the depression formed around each tree

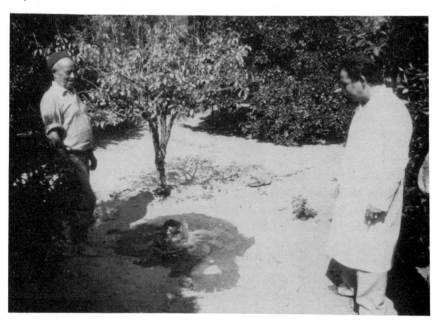

within the microbiological guidelines recommended by a WHO Scientific Group for wastewater reuse in agriculture.

Wastewater is distributed to farmers by local Agricultural Development Authorities, which are responsible to the Ministry of Agriculture. These Authorities construct and maintain the wastewater distribution system (pipelines, pumping stations, storage reservoirs, etc.), distribute the wastewater to the farmers according to an organized delivery schedule, and collect revenue. The farmers are responsible for on-farm distribution of the wastewater and pay 0.025 dinars (US$ 0.031) per m³ of wastewater to the Authorities by quarterly bills. The Authorities forbid the irrigation of crops eaten raw and have legal powers to enforce this restriction. Their personnel maintain regular contact with the farmers and ensure that the system is working properly.

3.2 Excreta use in agriculture

3.2.1 China

In China natural organic wastes are extensively used for soil fertilization. These wastes include excreta, domestic refuse, animal manure (principally from pigs and cows), crop residues and green manures such as *Azolla* and other aquatic plants. Urban nightsoil is collected and transported by cart, tractor and boat to rural areas. In 1981, 73 million tonnes of nightsoil and 73 million tonnes of refuse were produced in large- and medium-sized cities; of this, some 40 million tonnes were reused in agriculture and aquaculture. Treatment, although now becoming more common, is comparatively rare, with less than 5% of reused wastes being treated; composting is the most usual treatment process. Urban wastes that are not directly used in agriculture are generally disposed of in sanitary landfills which, when complete, are most commonly used for agricultural production (Zhongjie, 1986).

In the rural areas of China the wastes from some 800 million people are reused: the excreta usage rate is over 70% (Zhongjie, 1986). Animal manure is widely used—about 1.3 billion tons in 1981, as compared with 150 million tons of human excreta. Excreta are generally stored for four weeks before use, in order to destroy helminth eggs. Co-composting of human and animal excreta with crop residues is widely practised, as is biogas production, with subsequent use of the biogas slurry on the land. Nearly 2 billion tons of organic fertilizer are produced annually by these processes. Artificial fertilizers are used, but reliance on waste-derived organic fertilizers will continue because (FAO, 1977):

- there is 4000 years' experience of matching the various types of organic fertilizers to the local soils, and it will take time to develop an equivalent understanding of artificial fertilizers;

- artificial fertilizers are relatively expensive, whereas organic fertilizers are widely available at little or no financial cost;

- farmers generally prefer organic fertilizers because they increase the humus content of the soil and so improve its structure and water retention;

- Chinese soils are generally more responsive to nitrogen than to phosphate, and to phosphate than to potassium; most soils are not deficient in micronutrients because of the long-term application of organic fertilizers; and

- the construction of artificial fertilizer factories is very expensive, and the development of a fertilizer industry has to be a gradual process, depending upon the availability of internal resources rather than upon imports.

The bulk of human and animal excreta and excreta-derived compost is generally applied during land preparation before planting, and is ploughed or harrowed into the soil. The rate of application varies according to the soil, crop and season, but application rates for composts are usually 100–300 t/ha per year, and for liquid nightsoil 20–30 t/ha at each application. The principal criteria used to determine the exact application rate in any one case are: the quantity of available nutrients, especially nitrogen; prevention of any inhibition of germination and seedling growth; and the amount that can be effectively deposited on or incorporated into the land.

Experiments have shown that even relatively low application rates (15–40 t/ha per year) of excreta-derived compost can substantially increase crop yields (FAO, 1977): maize, 29%; millet, 48%; potato, 89%; sorghum, 85%; soya bean, 23%; sugar-beet, 26%; wheat, 39%.

3.2.2 Guatemala

Following the 1976 earthquake, the Centro Mesoamericano de Estudios sobre Tecnologia Apropriada (CEMAT) has been developing simple rural sanitation technologies that are compatible with agricultural reuse. A modification of the Vietnamese double-vault composting toilet, known as the Dry Alkaline Fertilizer Family (DAFF) latrine (or Letrina Abonera Seca Familiar, LASF), has been developed and is now fairly well established in some parts of rural Guatemala (Cacares, 1981; Strauss, 1986a). The DAFF latrine is an above-ground facility, comprising two alternating vaults constructed in brickwork and a simple bamboo superstructure. Faeces only are deposited in the vaults, and urine is collected separately. Ash from wood-burning stoves is added to the vault at least daily and preferably after each use. When one vault is full (usually after 4–6 months), it is sealed and the other vault is put into service. When the second vault is full, the first is emptied (see Figure 3.3) and its contents kept for application to the land immediately before planting or sowing. Urine, after dilution with water, is used for plant watering.

After 4–6 months of anaerobic mesophilic composting in the vault the contents are transformed into a dry, odourless material with a crumbly soil-like consistency. The organic matter content is 3–10%

Figure 3.3 A DAFF latrine in Guatemala being emptied
The digested excreta is then applied to the land

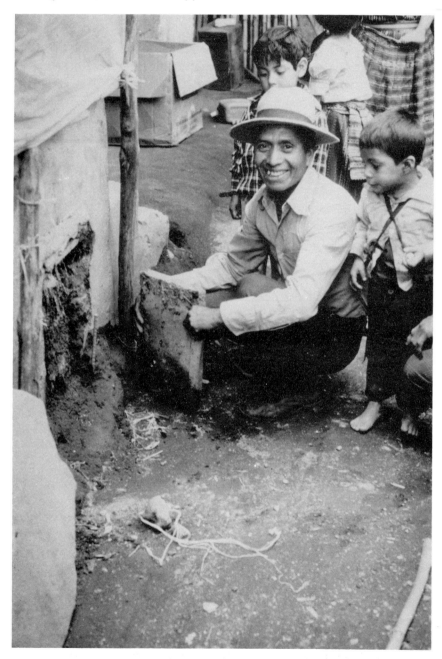

with 0.3–1.1% total nitrogen, 150–410 mg/kg of total phosphorus and 7000–7600 mg/kg of total potassium; the pH is high because of the large quantities of ash added and in the range 9.8–11.2. Coliform counts are reasonably low, generally less than 4000 per gram (wet weight), and helminth eggs are fewer than 8500 per gram with a viability of less than 30%. This microbiological quality is considered safe for reuse (Zandstra, 1986).

Local farmers regard the DAFF latrine as useful because:

- it provides a readily available, low-cost fertilizer and soil conditioner which "noticeably" improves crop yields (quantitative yield data are not available); and

- it is an odourless household sanitation facility that avoids the need for indiscriminate defecation in the fields.

Occasionally insufficient quantities of ash are available and sometimes soil or lime is added instead of, or in addition to, the ash in order to keep the vault contents at a moisture content of around 50%.

The DAFF latrine costs about US$ 70 to construct, and there is an additional cost of US$ 70 per latrine to cover training and promotion. The compost produced is worth US$ 12 per 50-kg bag and, as a family of five can produce 10 bags annually, the latrine costs can be recovered in little over a year.

3.2.3 India

Agricultural use of nightsoil is common in India, especially in areas near towns and cities (Strauss, 1986d). Nightsoil from bucket latrines is taken manually to transfer stations, from where it is transported by cart or truck to trenching grounds or delivered directly to the farmers. The nightsoil is sometimes stored in pits before use, but much is used without any treatment. Some is applied to the field before planting, and in other cases it is applied while the crops are growing. In some cities, such as Greater Calcutta, Kanpur and Lucknow, nightsoil and municipal refuse are co-composted. In the Calcutta region the compost is sold to farmers at an average rate of Rs 2.50 (US$ 0.23) per tonne; demand for the compost is often high, and it is frequently sold before it is fully matured. Strauss (1986d) gives the following quotation describing the nightsoil trenching and composting operations in Greater Calcutta:

> In the majority of cases the trenching or composting ground is not well suited for the purpose. Either they are low lying areas subject to flooding

in the monsoon, or the land is inadequate being mostly filled up, or inhabitation has come up all round or there is no approach to the ground. Neither composting, nor trenching is practised in a scientific way. Generally the nightsoil is emptied into pits of any size and no coverage by ash or mud is given. Once filled they are fully exposed to fly breeding etc. In some cases they even look like cesspools being filled with water during the rains. Similarly, composting also is not practised in a scientific way. Refuse and nightsoil are simply dumped in any fashion and in any proportion. In some municipalities it was even observed that nightsoil is emptied into water bodies within the trenching ground and this water is being used for bathing and washing etc. Workers are generally immunised but no other protection is provided to them. Municipal workers involved in the operation of disposal grounds are mostly ignorant about the technicalities involved.

In many of the excreta use schemes in India there is little apparent control, and the actual health risks are probably high (see Section 4.3). The current programmes for the replacement of bucket latrines with twin-pit pour-flush toilets will mean a gradual reduction in the quantity of fresh nightsoil available for agricultural use and a concurrent increase in the quantity of safe latrine sludge.

3.2.4 United States of America

The city of Kearney, Nebraska, has a population of 25 000 and produces some 3000–4000 tonnes of sludge annually at its wastewater treatment plant (Anon., 1986). Before 1984, this sludge was dewatered to 20% solids and transported 25 km for landfill disposal at an abandoned airbase. Now it is taken just 0.4 km to a local farm for co-composting with feedlot manure. The sludge and manure are mixed in the proportion 1:2, composted in mechanically turned windrows for five weeks, and stockpiled for four to five months. The compost is then spread on 1200 ha of agricultural land (used for raising corn) twice a year in spring and autumn, at the rate of 7.5–10 t/ha. It contains sufficient phosphorus and potassium, but the sandy soil requires the addition of supplemental nitrogen. The retail value of the nutrients in the compost is high: some $28 per tonne (see Table 3.4). The water retention of the soil is better because of its increased humus content, and no artificial fertilizers (other than the supplemental nitrogen) are required. Although this case study describes only a small-scale operation, its potential for replication in an intensely agricultural state is clearly very high.

Table 3.4 Retail value of nutrients in composted sludge and feedlot manure at Kearney, Nebraska

Nutrient	Concentration in compost (kg/t)	Cost (US¢/kg)	Value (US$/t compost)
Nitrogen	6.4	59.4	3.80
Phosphorus	7.3	66.0	4.82
Potassium	30.9	33.0	10.20
Sulfur	2.3	50.6	1.16
Zinc	0.1	330.0	0.33
Calcium	11.8	1.8	0.21
Magnesium	3.2	5.5	0.18
Iron	1.8	330.0	5.94
Manganese	0.1	163.0	0.16
Copper	0.2	748.0	1.50
		Total value: US$	28.30

3.3 Wastewater and excreta use in aquaculture

3.3.1 India

There are more than 132 wastewater-fertilized fish-pond systems in India, covering an area of 120 km²; most are located in West Bengal. The largest of these is the Calcutta wastewater fisheries, and this system is also the largest example of wastewater-based aquaculture in the world (Bose, 1944; Edwards, 1985; Strauss, 1986d).

Raw wastewater from Calcutta is conveyed in two 27-km canals to the North and South Salt Lake fisheries constructed on the wetlands of East Calcutta. The canals feed into a complex system of secondary and tertiary canals, from which wastewater is fed into the fish-ponds (see Figure 3.4). There are some 4400 ha of ponds, which are stocked with Indian major carp and tilapia. The ponds are emptied each year in February to remove the bottom mud and any vegetation, and refilled with partially diluted wastewater 6 to 8 weeks later. After a period of 2–3 weeks to permit the development of phytoplankton, the ponds are stocked with fish and wastewater is slowly fed into them for 5–10 days each month; this slow rate of wastewater introduction avoids deoxygenation of the fish-ponds. The fish attain marketable size in 5–6 months, and mean annual yields for the North and South fisheries are approximately 1400 and 1000 kg/ha respectively.

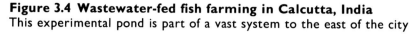

Figure 3.4 Wastewater-fed fish farming in Calcutta, India
This experimental pond is part of a vast system to the east of the city

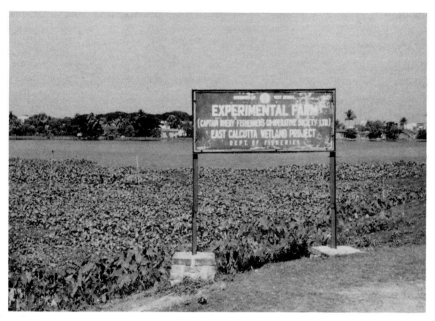

Some of the fish-ponds are leased from the City of Calcutta, some are privately owned and a few are run as cooperatives; they provide employment for the local people at a rate of 7.5 persons per hectare. The fish are caught at dawn in traditional drag nets and sold at local auctions, from where they go to the Calcutta markets; by 0700 h most of the day's catch has been sold. The fish-ponds supply 10–20% of the fish consumed in Greater Calcutta.

Trematode infections are not endemic in West Bengal, and total coliform counts in the fish-ponds are around 100–1000 per 100 ml. This, together with the fact that the fish are consumed well cooked (usually by deep frying), indicates a low potential risk for disease transmission.

3.3.2 Indonesia

The fertilization of fish-ponds with excreta is mainly practised in southeastern West Java. In the four regencies (administrative areas) of Bandung, Ciamis, Garut and Tasikmalaya, where this practice is most common and which have a population of nearly 8 million, some 33 000 tonnes of fish, predominantly common carp and Java and Nile

Figure 3.5 An overhanging latrine in Java, Indonesia
Excreta fall into the pond and fertilize fish production. The bamboo pipes in the foreground bring water for bathing and washing from other ponds

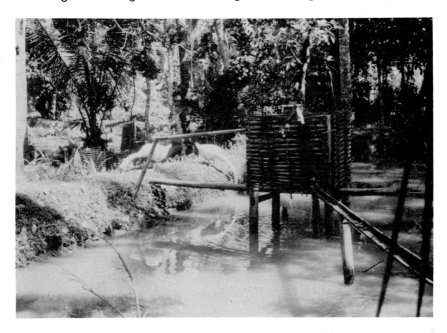

tilapia, are produced annually in approximately 10 000 ha of ponds (B. Abisudjak, personal communication).

Strauss (1986c) describes excreta-based fish culture in the village of Cikoneng, which has a population of 3900 and is located 20 km south-east of Bandung. Cikoneng is a typical "pond village": the natural surface drainage from rivulets and streams discharges into 5 ha of ponds (the average pond size is 590 m²), into which local run-off and water from paddy fields are also directed through bamboo gutters and pipes. The ponds are interconnected, and water flows from the upper to the lower ponds. The ponds are used for washing and bathing by all except the richer families who have their own well, and overhanging latrines (Figure 3.5) are constructed in the ponds for excreta disposal and direct fertilization of the fish. Rice bran and chicken manure are also used by some families for fertilization. The ponds are completely drained once a year, and all the fish are caught and sold. Annual fish yields are in the range 1600–2800 kg/ha. The bottom mud is removed and used in the local rice fields as a soil conditioner and fertilizer. Fish are also caught once a week for local consumption after cooking. In some ponds, water spinach is also grown, and this is eaten as a cooked vegetable. Diarrhoeal disease is not a major health problem in the village, with around only one episode per person per year. Faecal coliform counts in the fish ponds range between 10^4 and 10^5 per 100 ml. Trematode infections (clonorchiasis, fasciolopsiasis and schistosomiasis) are absent. The practice of fish-pond fertilization with raw excreta does not appear to promote any significant excess transmission of excreta-related disease.

4
Public health aspects

In developing countries excreta-related diseases are common, and excreta and wastewater contain correspondingly high concentrations of excreted pathogens. It is important to understand the transmission routes of these diseases and the health risk factors involved, in order to design and implement or modify excreta and wastewater use schemes that do not result in any increased transmission of these diseases.

4.1 Excreta-related infections

The infections in question are communicable diseases whose causative agents (pathogenic viruses, bacteria, protozoa and helminths) escape from the bodies of infected persons in their excreta, eventually reaching other people, whom they enter via either the mouth (for example when contaminated vegetables are eaten) or the skin (as in the case of hookworm and schistosomiasis). There are 30 known excreta-related infections of public health importance, and these may be conveniently grouped into five categories according to environmental transmission characteristics and pathogen properties (see Table 4.1).

Category I infections are caused by excreted viruses and protozoa and the helminths *Enterobius vermicularis* (pinworm or threadworm) and *Hymenolepis nana* (dwarf tapeworm). These pathogens are infective immediately on excretion ("non-latent") and have a low median infective dose. Transmission of these diseases occurs predominantly in the immediate domestic environment, especially when low standards of personal hygiene prevail, although survival times of excreted viruses and protozoa may be long enough to pose a health risk in excreta and wastewater use schemes (see Section 4.2).

The pathogens causing Category II infections are the excreted bacteria. Like the causative agents of Category I infections they are infective immediately on excretion. They are moderately persistent and can multiply outside their host, for example in food or milk. They are also very commonly transmitted in the immediate domestic environment, but their greater persistence means that they can

Table 4.1 Environmental classification of excreted infections

Category and epidemiological features	Infection	Environmental transmission focus	Major control measure
I. Non-latent; low infective dose	Amoebiasis Balantidiasis Enterobiasis Enteroviral infections Giardiasis Hymenolepiasis Hepatitis A Rotavirus infection	Personal Domestic	Domestic water supply Health education Improved housing Provision of toilets
II. Non-latent; medium or high infective dose; moderately persistent; able to multiply	*Campylobacter* infection Cholera Pathogenic *Escherichia coli* infection Salmonellosis Shigellosis Typhoid Yersiniosis	Personal Domestic Water Crop	Domestic water supply Health education Improved housing Provision of toilets Treatment of excreta before discharge or reuse
III. Latent and persistent; no intermediate host	Ascariasis Hookworm infection Strongyloidiasis Trichuriasis	Yard Field Crop	Provision of toilets Treatment of excreta before land application

Category	Disease	Transmission	Control measures
IV. Latent and persistent; cow or pig as intermediate host	Taeniasis	Yard Field Fodder	Provisions of toilets Treatment of excreta before land application Cooking, meat inspection
V. Latent and persistent; aquatic intermediate host(s)	Clonorchiasis Diphyllobothriasis Fascioliasis Fasciolopsiasis Gastrodiscoidiasis Heterophyiasis Metagonimiasis Opisthorchiasis Paragonimiasis Schistosomiasis	Water	Provision of toilets Treatment of excreta before discharge Control of animal reservoirs Control of intermediate hosts Cooking of water plants and fish Reducing water contact

Source: Feachem et al. (1983).

survive longer transmission routes and therefore they can, and do, pose real health risks in excreta and wastewater use schemes. There are well documented cases of, for example, cholera epidemics caused by the irrigation of vegetable crops with untreated wastewater.

Infections of Categories III to V are caused by excreted helminths, which all require a period of time after excretion to become infective to humans. This period of latency occurs in soil, in water or in an intermediate host; most of the helminths are environmentally persistent, with survival times usually ranging from several weeks to several years. Excreta and wastewater use schemes are important mechanisms for transmission of many of these diseases, and a major environmental measure for their control is the effective treatment of excreta, wastewater and wastewater-derived sludges before use (see Section 7).

The diseases in Category III are caused by the soil-transmitted intestinal nematodes that require no intermediate host. The most important of these are the human roundworm (*Ascaris lumbricoides*), the hookworms (*Ancylostoma duodenale* and *Necator americanus*) and the human whipworm (*Trichuris trichiura*). They are all readily transmitted by the agricultural use of raw or insufficiently treated excreta and wastewater; indeed, of all excreted pathogens these cause the greatest public health concern in agricultural use schemes (see Section 4.3).

Category IV infections are caused by the cow and pig tapeworms, *Taenia saginata* and *T. solium*, respectively. For their successful transmission viable eggs must be ingested by a cow or pig; a potential route for the transmission of these diseases is the irrigation of pasture with wastewater.

The infections in Category V are all water-based helminthic infections. The pathogens require one or two intermediate aquatic hosts, the first of which is a snail, in which huge asexual multiplication of the pathogen occurs, and the second (if there is one) either a fish or an aquatic macrophyte. Many of these helminths have a limited geographical distribution (see Feachem et al., 1983), and it is only in endemic areas that their transmission is promoted by the aquacultural use of raw or insufficiently treated excreta and wastewater, together with the practice of eating raw or inadequately cooked fish and aquatic vegetables. Agricultural use is not relevant, except in so far as all irrigation schemes may facilitate the transmission of schistosomiasis.

4.2 Health risks

4.2.1 Actual and potential risks

For the agricultural or aquacultural use of excreta and wastewater to pose an *actual* risk to health requires *all* of the following to occur:

(a) *either* an infective dose of an excreted pathogen reaches the field or pond, *or* the pathogen multiplies in the field or pond to form an infective dose;

(b) the infective dose reaches a human host;

(c) the host becomes infected; and

(d) the infection causes disease or further transmission.

The risk remains a *potential* risk if only (a), or (a) and (b), or (a), (b) and (c) occur, but not (d).

Even if there is an actual risk involved, the agricultural or aquacultural use of excreta or wastewater will be of public health importance only if it causes a measurable excess incidence or prevalence of disease or intensity of infection. Epidemiological studies are needed to determine whether this is the case (see Section 4.3).

The sequence of events required for an actual health risk to be posed is summarized in Figure 4.1, together with the pathogen-host properties and interactions that influence each step in the sequence. If the sequence is broken at any point, the potential risks cannot combine to constitute an actual risk. This is the rationale behind the various methods of public health protection discussed in Section 7.

4.2.2. Risk factors

There is ample evidence (Feachem et al., 1983) that excreta and wastewater may — and, especially in developing countries, usually do — contain high concentrations of excreted pathogens, and that many of these pathogens can survive in these materials for some time and can also withstand most conventional treatment processes. They can thus arrive at the field or pond in large enough numbers for human infection to be theoretically possible. The only way that this can be prevented from happening is to remove or kill the pathogens before they reach the field or pond. However, even if sufficient pathogens do reach the field or pond, infection occurs only if an

Figure 4.1 Pathogen-host properties influencing the sequence of events between the presence of a pathogen in excreta or wastewater and measurable human disease attributable to excreta or wastewater use

EXCRETED LOAD

- latency
- multiplication
- persistence
- treatment survival

INFECTIVE DOSE APPLIED TO LAND/WATER

- persistence
- intermediate host
- type of use practice
- type of human exposure

INFECTIVE DOSE REACHES HUMAN HOST

- human behaviour
- pattern of human immunity

RISKS OF INFECTION AND DISEASE

- alternative routes of transmission

PUBLIC HEALTH IMPORTANCE OF EXCRETA AND WASTEWATER USE

From Blum & Feachem (1985), reproduced by permission of the International Reference Centre for Waste Disposal.

infective dose is received by a susceptible host, and this depends on the following factors (Blum & Feachem, 1985):

- the survival time of the pathogen in soil, on crops, in fish or in water;

- the presence, for Category IV and V infections, of the required intermediate host or hosts;

- the mode and frequency of excreta or wastewater application;

- the type of crop to which the excreta or wastewater is applied; and

- the nature of exposure of the human host to the contaminated soil, water, crop or fish.

Pathogen survival

The extensive literature on the survival times of excreted pathogens in soil and on crop surfaces has been reviewed by Feachem et al. (1983) and Strauss (1985). There are wide variations in reported survival times, which reflect both strain variation and differing climatic factors as well as different analytical techniques. None the less it is possible to summarize current knowledge on pathogen survival in soil and on crops in warm climates (20–30 °C) as shown in Table 4.2. Pathogen survival in excreta- and wastewater-enriched ponds is similar to that in waste stabilization ponds (see Section 7.2). Bacterial and viral numbers may be expected to decrease by only 1–3 orders of magnitude, depending on the available dilution, hydraulic retention time and climatic factors; helminth eggs and protozoal

Table 4.2. Survival times of selected excreted pathogens in soil and on crop surfaces at 20–30 °C

Pathogen	Survival time (days)	
	In soil	On crops
Viruses		
Enteroviruses[a]	< 100 but usually < 20	< 60 but usually < 15
Bacteria		
Faecal coliforms	< 70 but usually < 20	< 30 but usually < 15
Salmonella spp.	< 70 but usually < 20	< 30 but usually < 15
Vibrio cholerae	< 20 but usually < 10	< 5 but usually < 2
Protozoa		
Entamoeba histolytica cysts	< 20 but usually < 10	< 10 but usually < 2
Helminths		
Ascaris lumbricoides eggs	Many months	< 60 but usually < 30
Hookworm larvae	< 90 but usually < 30	< 30 but usually < 10
Taenia saginata eggs	Many months	< 60 but usually < 30
Trichuris trichiura eggs	Many months	< 60 but usually < 30

[a] Includes poliovirus, echovirus, and coxsackievirus.

From Feachem et al. (1983), reproduced by permission of the World Bank.

cysts will settle to the bottom of the pond where they may remain viable for a long time.

The available evidence indicates that almost all excreted pathogens can survive in soil and ponds for a sufficient length of time to pose potential risks to farm and pond workers (see Figure 4.2). Pathogen survival on crop surfaces is much shorter than that in soil, as the pathogens are less well protected from the harsh effects of sunlight and desiccation. In some cases, however, survival times can be long enough to pose potential risks to crop handlers and consumers, especially when they exceed the length of crop (mainly vegetable) growing cycles (Figure 4.3). The situation is similar for those who handle and consume fish and aquatic macrophytes.

Intermediate hosts

Irrigation of pasture with wastewater that contains viable *Taenia saginata* eggs will induce bovine cysticercosis only if cows have access to the pasture while the eggs are still viable. An interval of at least 14 days between irrigation and grazing is therefore recommended and, in some countries, obligatory. Education of farmers and enforcement of regulations are necessary additional control measures. In the case of pig tapeworm, pigs become infected in practice only if they have direct access to human faeces (which they readily consume), and excreta fertilization and wastewater irrigation of crops do not generally promote any significant disease transmission.

In the case of Category V infections, the secondary intermediate aquatic host — a fish or aquatic plant — is the desired aquacultural product, and infection occurs only if a viable egg reaches the pond, if there are suitable snail hosts in the pond and if the secondary host is eaten raw or insufficiently cooked. These "aquacultural diseases" occur only in certain restricted geographical areas of Asia, where these three factors are all present (see Section 4.4.3).

Mode and frequency of application

The way in which excreta or wastewater is applied to the land or pond, the interval between successive applications and the interval between the last application and harvesting all affect the likely degree of crop contamination and the environmental dispersion of excreted pathogens. Strategies to minimize these effects are discussed in Section 7.4.

Figure 4.2 Pathogen survival in soil compared with vegetable growth periods in warm climates

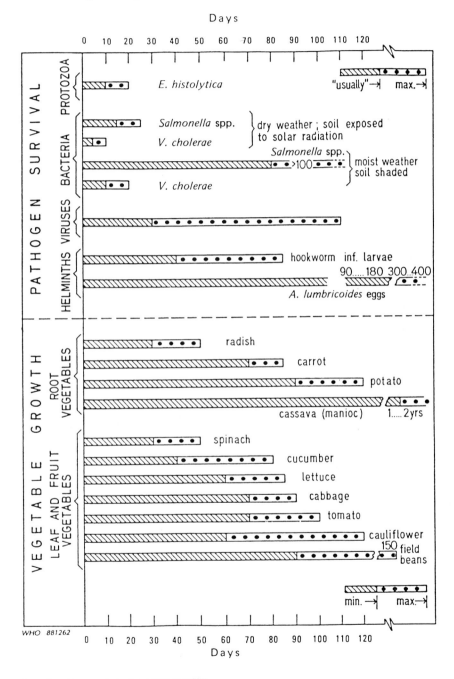

WHO 881262

Reproduced by permission from Strauss (1985).

Figure 4.3 Pathogen survival on crops compared with vegetable growth periods in warm climates

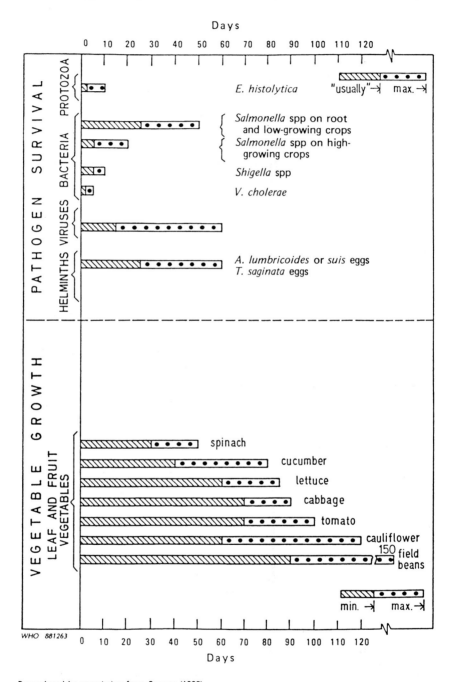

Reproduced by permission from Strauss (1985).

Type of crop and type of exposure

The production of agricultural and aquacultural crops intended for human consumption poses potential risks to farm or pond workers, to those who handle the products and to those who consume them. If the products are fodder crops, farm workers and those who consume the resulting meat or milk are at potential risk; in the case of industrial products (for example, sugar-beet, fishmeal) only farm or pond workers and product handlers are subjected to risk. In the case of sprinkler irrigation, people living near the irrigated fields, who are at potential risk from pathogens present in wind-dispersed aerosol droplets, form an additional exposure group.

The greatest risk is associated with crops eaten raw, for example salad crops, especially if they are root crops (such as radishes) or grow close to the soil (for instance, lettuces). Pathogen survival times can be greater than the crop growing time, so that contamination is highly likely unless the excreta or wastewater is treated to a very high standard (see Section 7.2).

Host immunity

Significant host immunity occurs only with the viral diseases and some bacterial diseases (for example typhoid). The role of immunity is most noticeable in the case of viral infections where infection at an early age is very common (even in communities with high standards of personal hygiene), with the result that the adult population is largely immune to the disease and frequently also to infection.

Human behaviour

Adequate standards of personal and food hygiene and, in the case of occupational exposure, the wearing of protective clothing and foot-wear can protect against infection even in situations where the risk of infection would otherwise be extremely high. Health education is needed to alter certain behavioural patterns. However, this is a long-term solution and may not be at all effective in modifying certain cultural preferences, for example the eating of raw fish. Sociocultural aspects of excreta and wastewater use are discussed further in Section 5.

Alternative routes of pathogen transmission

The factors outlined above determine the potential health risks associated with excreta and wastewater use. The relative importance of such risks depends on the existence of any alternative routes by which the excreted pathogens reach those at risk. If there are many such alternative routes, excreta and wastewater use may not pose a significant additional risk. Conversely, if there are no such routes, excreta and wastewater use is entirely responsible for the risk induced.

These two situations may be illustrated by considering the inhabitants of a wealthy, modern city and those of a poor, traditional village who both consume vegetables fertilized with the villagers' excreta. Let us suppose that the standards of personal and environmental hygiene are very high in the city, but very low in the village. Then the only (or almost the only) exposure of the city inhabitants to excreted pathogens is via the vegetables. For the villagers, however, this transmission route will be only one of many, and not necessarily the most important, since the high level of faecal contamination of their immediate environment is likely to give rise to much more direct exposure and consequent infection and disease. Thus, preventing consumption of the vegetables in the city would be an effective control strategy, but similar measures in the village would probably have little if any effect on the disease transmission rate.

4.3 Epidemiological evidence

The actual public health importance of excreta or wastewater use can be assessed only by determining whether it results in an incidence, prevalence or intensity of disease measurably in excess of that which occurs in its absence. If it does not, its public health importance is negligible. On the other hand, if it does, the magnitude of its importance will depend upon the balance between the public health significance of the measured excess incidence, prevalence or intensity and its public health benefits. Benefits may include improved community nutrition resulting from increased food consumption, for instance.

An epidemiological study is required to determine whether excreta or wastewater use in a particular context results in a measurable excess incidence, prevalence or intensity of disease. Such studies are methodologically difficult but have no substitute if actual — as opposed to potential — health risks are to be assessed. Despite the fact that there have been relatively few well designed epidemiological studies on excreta and wastewater use, it is possible to draw certain conclusions from the evidence currently available. This is easiest in the case of wastewater irrigation, for which the evidence is greatest;

there is much less information about agricultural use of excreta and aquacultural use of wastewater and excreta.

4.3.1 Agricultural use of wastewater

Shuval et al. (1986) have rigorously reviewed all the available epidemiological studies conducted on the agricultural use of waste-water. Their principal conclusions can be summarized as follows:

- Crop irrigation with untreated wastewater causes significant excess infection with intestinal nematodes in both consumers (Figure 4.4) and farm workers (Figure 4.5); the latter, especially if

Figure 4.4 Relationship between *Ascaris*-positive stool samples in the population of western Jerusalem and the availability of vegetables and salad crops irrigated with raw waste-water in Jerusalem, 1935–1982

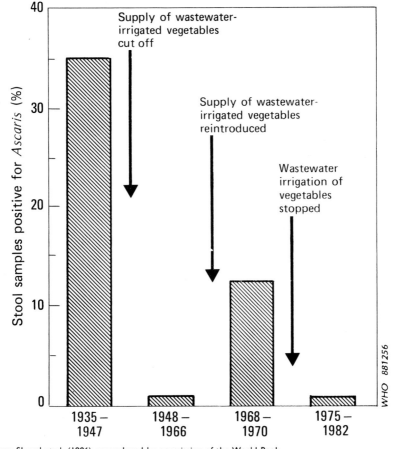

From Shuval et al. (1986), reproduced by permission of the World Bank.

Figure 4.5 Prevalence of hookworm and *Ascaris* infections in sewage farm workers and control groups in various regions of India

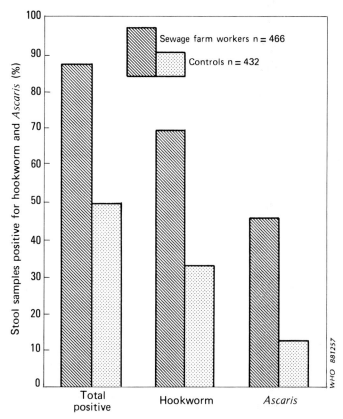

From Shuval et al. (1986), reproduced by permission of the World Bank.

they work barefoot in the fields, are likely to have more intense infections, particularly of hookworms, than those not working in wastewater-irrigated fields.

- Crop irrigation with treated wastewater[1] does not lead to excess intestinal nematode infection among field workers or consumers (Figure 4.6).

- Cholera, and probably also typhoid, can be effectively transmitted by the irrigation of vegetables with untreated wastewater (see Box 4.1).

---

[1] "Treated wastewater" here refers to conventional treatment, that is primary sedimentation, biological treatment (trickling filters or activated sludge) and secondary sedimentation. Conventional effluents contain few helminth ova or protozoan cysts but have high concentrations of faecal bacteria and viruses (see Section 7).

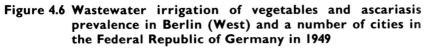

Figure 4.6 Wastewater irrigation of vegetables and ascariasis prevalence in Berlin (West) and a number of cities in the Federal Republic of Germany in 1949

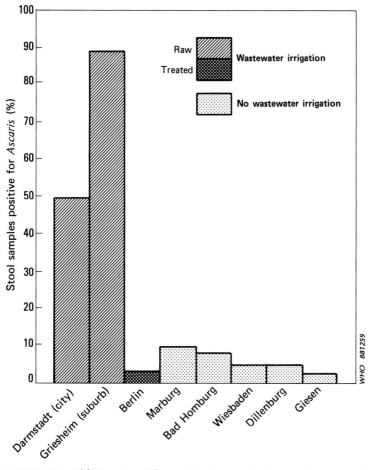

Raw wastewater was used for irrigation in Darmstadt and conventionally treated wastewater (primary sedimentation, biofiltration and secondary sedimentation) in Berlin (West).

From Shuval et al. (1986), reproduced by permission of the World Bank.

- Cattle grazing on pasture irrigated with raw wastewater may become infected with *Cysticercus bovis* (the larval stage of the beef tapeworm *Taenia saginata*), but there is little evidence for actual risk of human infection.

- There is limited evidence that the health of people living near fields irrigated with raw wastewater may be negatively affected, either directly by contact with the soil or indirectly through

Box 4.1 The 1970 Jerusalem cholera epidemic

The cholera epidemic that occurred in Jerusalem in August and September 1970 was the first occasion on which credible epidemiological evidence was obtained for the transmission of an excreted bacterial infection by wastewater-irrigated vegetables.

In the summer of 1970 numerous cases of cholera were reported in the countries adjacent to Israel. Three cases of cholera appeared in Jerusalem on August 20. The outbreak reached a peak of 59 cases in the week of September 13–19. All known acute cases were investigated in detail: there was little evidence of secondary contact — no infections were found in family groups or among co-workers — and there was no spread to other Israeli cities, even though Jerusalem remained open for normal commerce and tourism. It thus appeared that a common-source epidemic was occurring.

Routine bacteriological monitoring of the city's water supply indicated zero coliform counts; all milk and dairy products were pasteurized under strict laboratory quality control; general sanitation within the city was high — there were few or no exposed excreta and a low housefly population.

The most likely common source appeared to be the salad crops and vegetables grown in the Kidron and Refaim valleys adjacent to the city, where fields were irrigated with the city's raw wastewater.

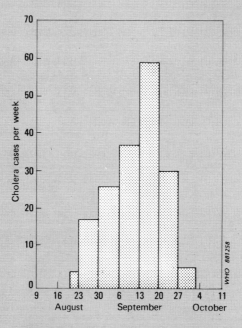

Weekly distribution of cholera cases in Jerusalem, August–September 1970 (*n* = 176). Irrigation of vegetables and salad crops with raw wastewater was stopped by the authorities during the week beginning September 13.

(Box 4.1 continued)

Their purchase was often mentioned by those who contracted the disease, and in several cases the only family member who became ill was the one who had consumed these products.

An intensive programme of sampling and testing for *Vibrio cholerae* in the wastewater in the city's main outfall sewers, in the soil on the wastewater-irrigated fields and on vegetables growing there and on sale in local markets was initiated. During the epidemic 18% of wastewater samples were positive for *V. cholerae*, and serological examination showed that the *V. cholerae* isolates were the same serotype as that found in the vast majority of the clinical cases; no *V. cholerae* were found in wastewater after the epidemic. Cholera vibrios and phages were also detected in the wastewater-irrigated soil and on vegetables grown there and on sale in local markets. Subsequent laboratory studies showed that *V. cholerae* could survive in wastewater, on soil and on crop surfaces for long enough to make this mode of transmission possible.

The Israeli health authorities ordered the cessation of the growing and marketing of wastewater-irrigated crops; harvested crops were confiscated and those still growing destroyed during September 15–20. The epidemic rapidly subsided and the last clinical case was detected some 12 days later.

It is now clear that the 1970 cholera epidemic in Jerusalem was initiated by imported clinical or subclinical cases, and that the main pathway for the secondary spread of the disease was through wastewater-irrigated vegetables.

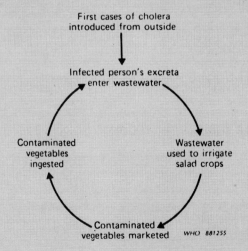

First cases of cholera
introduced from outside

Infected person's excreta
enter wastewater

Contaminated
vegetables
ingested

Wastewater
used to irrigate
salad crops

Contaminated
vegetables marketed   WHO 881255

Hypothesized cycle of transmission of *Vibrio cholerae* from first cholera cases or carriers introduced from outside Jerusalem, through wastewater-irrigated vegetables, back to residents in the city.

Source: Shuval et al. (1986)

contact with farm labourers. In communities with high standards of personal hygiene such negative impacts are usually restricted to an excess incidence of benign gastroenteritis, often of viral etiology, although there may also be an excess of bacterial infections.

- Sprinkler irrigation with treated wastewater[1] may promote the aerosol transmission of excreted viruses, but disease transmission is likely to be rare in practice since most people have high levels of immunity to the viral diseases endemic in their community.

From these findings it is clear that, when untreated wastewater is used for crop irrigation, intestinal nematodes and bacteria present high actual risk and the viruses little or no actual risk (see Table 4.3). The actual risks of protozoal infection are not yet well established — insufficient epidemiological data are available — but no study has shown that waste reuse causes additional risk. It is also clear that treatment of wastewater is a very effective method of safeguarding public health.

4.3.2 Agricultural use of excreta

Blum & Feachem (1985) have extensively reviewed the existing epidemiological literature on the transmission of disease associated with the fertilization of crops with excreta. Many of the studies reviewed are from China and Japan where this practice is, or was, common. Their conclusions are very similar to those of Shuval et al. (1986) for crop irrigation, and can be summarized as follows:

- Crop fertilization with raw excreta causes excess infection with intestinal nematodes in both consumers and field workers.

- There is evidence that excreta treatment reduces the transmission of nematode infection.

- The fertilization of rice paddies with excreta may lead to excess schistosomiasis infection among rice farmers.

---

[1] "Treated wastewater" here refers to conventional treatment, that is primary sedimentation, biological treatment (trickling filters or activated sludge) and secondary sedimentation. Conventional effluents contain few helminth ova or protozoan cysts but have high concentrations of faecal bacteria and viruses (see Section 7).

Table 4.3 Relative health risks from use of untreated excreta and wastewater in agriculture and aquaculture

Class of pathogen	Relative excess frequency of infection or disease
Intestinal nematodes: Ascaris Trichuris Ancylostoma Necator	High
Bacterial infections: bacterial diarrhoeas (e.g. cholera, typhoid)	Lower
Viral infections: viral diarrhoeas hepatitis A	Least
Trematode and cestode infections: schistosomiasis clonorchiasis taeniasis	From high to nil, depending upon the particular excreta use practice and local circumstances

- Cattle may become infected with *Cysticercus bovis* but are unlikely to contract salmonellosis.

4.3.3 Aquacultural use

Three potential health risks are associated with the aquacultural use of excreta and wastewater (Feachem et al., 1983):

- passive transference of excreted pathogens by fish and cultured aquatic macrophytes;

- transmission of trematodes whose life cycles involve fish and aquatic macrophytes (principally *Clonorchis sinensis* and *Fasciolopsis buski*); and

- transmission of schistosomiasis.

Blum & Feachem (1985) also reviewed the available epidemiological studies on excreta use in aquaculture. They found only one study that considered actual health risks associated with the passive transference of excreted pathogens, and the results of this were inconclusive because of the epidemiological methodology employed. They found none dealing with occupational exposure leading to schistosomiasis. With respect to trematode infections they found that fertilization of ponds with excreta was important in the transmission of these diseases but that so too was incidental faecal pollution of other local water bodies and ponds not purposefully fertilized with excreta.

4.4 Microbiological quality criteria

The epidemiological evidence briefly reviewed above clearly indicates that certain current excreta and wastewater use practices can result in actual health risks to certain exposure groups (for example, nematode and bacterial infections). In some cases (viral disease transmission by wastewater irrigation) the evidence indicates that there is no risk of excess disease and in others (bacterial disease risks in aquacultural use) no unequivocal evidence is available. The existing epidemiological data base needs of course to be improved. Despite its limitations, however, it can be usefully combined with a realistic appraisal of potential health risks to provide a reasonable basis for the development of microbiological quality criteria for treated excreta and wastewater intended for agricultural and aquacultural use.

The engineer who designs an excreta or wastewater treatment plant needs to know the extent to which excreted pathogens must be removed. The strict epidemiological answer is that the degree of treatment required is that which prevents excess disease transmission. This is not a helpful answer, however, because of the considerable uncertainty over minimal infective doses of many of the excreted pathogens, and because treatment efficiency is determined not by the residual concentration of pathogens (or pathogen indicators) in the treated wastes, but by the proportion removed. None the less, the design engineer needs a treatment product standard expressed in terms of the maximum permissible concentration(s) of specified organisms for each excreta and wastewater use practice. Microbiological quality criteria have been promulgated in several countries for wastewater intended for crop irrigation, but no criteria have yet been established for the quality of excreta used for crop fertilization or of excreta or wastewater for aquacultural use.

4.4.1 Wastewater quality for agricultural use

Historically, criteria[1] for the quality of wastewater for crop irrigation have been developed by borrowing from the water supply industry the concept of faecal indicator organisms. Coliform bacteria have long been used for this purpose and, while others exist, coliforms are still the indicator organism most commonly used despite the fact that not all of them are exclusively faecal. Non-faecal strains are of no use in assessing faecal pollution, and only the "faecal coliforms", which are indeed exclusively faecal in origin, can be used for this purpose. The term "total coliforms" is used to refer to an undifferentiated population of faecal and non-faecal types.

Wastewater quality guidelines and standards[1] are thus often expressed in terms of maximum permissible concentrations of total and/or faecal coliform bacteria. Since the faecal origin of wastewater is not in question, the implication is that these faecal indicator organisms can be used as pathogen indicators, and that there is at least a semiquantitative relationship between pathogen and indicator concentrations. In practice faecal coliforms can be used as reasonably reliable indicators of bacterial pathogens, as their environmental survival characteristics and rates of removal or die-off in treatment processes are broadly similar. Total coliforms are less reliable since, in warm climates especially, the proportion of non-faecal coliforms is often very high. Faecal coliforms are less effective as indicators of excreted viruses, and of very limited use for protozoa and helminths for which no reliable indicators exist.

Standards or guidelines for wastewater quality for crop irrigation generally specify both explicit standards (for example maximum coliform concentrations) and minimum treatment requirements (primary, secondary or tertiary) according to the class of crop to be irrigated (consumable, non-consumable). Standards developed 10–20 years ago tend to be very strict, as they were based on an evaluation of potential health risks associated with pathogen survival in wastewater, in soil and on crops, and on technical feasibility. The technology of choice for pathogen removal at that time (as judged by coliform removal) was effluent chlorination and, since this could easily achieve very low residual coliform concentrations, the maximum permissible coliform concentration was set correspondingly

---

[1] The scientific community develops, on the basis of the evidence available, quality *criteria*. These are used by such agencies as FAO and WHO to develop quality *guidelines*. These in turn can be used by governments to establish quality *standards* that can be enforced through laws and regulations in the country concerned.

low. For example, the 1968 California standards permit only 23 or 2.3 total coliforms per 100 ml, depending on the crop being irrigated (California State Department of Public Health, 1968); in 1973 a WHO Meeting of Experts noted that it was "technically feasible under field conditions to produce a sewage effluent containing not more than 100 coliform organisms per 100 ml" and that unrestricted irrigation of agricultural crops with such effluent was likely to produce only "a limited health risk" (World Health Organization, 1973). However, there is a wide variation in standards for wastewater use, as shown in Table 4.4.

Table 4.4 Examples of current microbiological standards for wastewater used for crop irrigation

Country	Restricted irrigation	Unrestricted irrigation
Oman	Maximum 23 TC/100 ml[a] Average <2.2 TC/100 ml Greenbelt irrigation only	Crop irrigation not permitted
Kuwait	<10 000 TC/100 ml	<100 TC/100 ml Not salad crops or strawberries
Saudi Arabia	Use of secondary effluent permitted for forage crops, field crops and vegetables which are processed and also for landscape irrigation	<2.2 TC/100 ml <50 FC/100 ml[b]
Tunisia	Fruit trees, forage crops and vegetables eaten cooked: — secondary treatment (including chlorination) — absence of *Vibrio cholerae* and salmonellae	No irrigation of vegetables eaten raw
Mexico	For recreational areas: <10 000 TC/100 ml <2 000 FC/100 ml	For vegetables eaten raw and fruits with possible soil contact: <1000 TC/100 ml
Peru	Treatment specified depending on reuse option	No irrigation of low-growing and root crops that may be eaten raw

[a] TC: total coliforms
[b] FC: faecal coliforms

Reproduced by permission from Strauss (1987).

Evaluation of the credible epidemiological evidence — that is, an appraisal of the actual, as opposed to potential, health risks (Section 4.3) — indicates that these standards may be unjustifiably restrictive. Moreover, design methods for waste stabilization ponds, which are generally the wastewater treatment system of first choice in developing countries (see Section 7.2), have been refined considerably during the past 10–20 years, so that any required level of pathogen removal can now be readily achieved with a very high degree of confidence. As a result of these considerations, a Meeting of Experts sponsored by the World Bank, the World Health Organization and the International Reference Centre for Waste Disposal (IRCWD) and held in Engelberg, Switzerland, in July 1985, recommended the guidelines shown in Table 4.5. A detailed explanation of the rationale for the "Engelberg" quality guidelines is given in Box 4.2 as the "Adelboden Statement."

Table 4.5 Tentative microbiological quality guidelines for treated wastewater reuse in agricultural irrigation

Note: In specific cases, the guidelines should be modified according to local epidemiological, sociocultural, and hydrogeological factors.

Reuse process	Intestinal nematodes[a] (arithmetic mean no. of viable eggs per litre)	Faecal coliforms (geometric mean no. per 100 ml)
Restricted irrigation[b] Irrigation of trees, industrial crops, fodder crops, fruit trees[c] and pasture[d]	$\leqslant 1$	not applicable
Unrestricted irrigation Irrigation of edible crops, sports fields, and public parks[e]	$\leqslant 1$	$\leqslant 1000$[f]

[a] *Ascaris, Trichuris* and hookworms.
[b] A minimum degree of treatment equivalent to at least a 1-day anaerobic pond followed by a 5-day facultative pond or its equivalent is required in all cases.
[c] Irrigation should cease two weeks before fruit is picked, and no fruit should be picked off the ground.
[d] Irrigation should cease two weeks before animals are allowed to graze.
[e] Local epidemiological factors may require a more stringent standard for public lawns, especially hotel lawns in tourist areas.
[f] When edible crops are always consumed well cooked, this recommendation may be less stringent.

Source: International Reference Centre for Waste Disposal (1985)

The Engelberg quality guidelines for restricted irrigation (trees, industrial and fodder crops, fruit trees and pasture) introduced for the first time an explicit helminth standard (<1 viable intestinal nematode egg per litre), which implies a very high degree of egg removal ($>99\%$). Its purpose is to protect the health of agricultural workers, who are at high risk from intestinal nematode infection. Wastewater complying with this guideline will contain few, if any, protozoan cysts so that field workers and consumers will also be protected from protozoal infections. Similarly, the wastewater will contain no (or, exceptionally, very few) *Taenia* eggs, so that grazing cattle will be protected from *Cysticercus bovis* and thus consumers also from beef tapeworm infection. There are several treatment options to achieve this quality, but the most appropriate in many cases will be a waste stabilization pond system comprising a 1–2-day anaerobic pond followed by a facultative pond and a maturation pond, each with a retention time of at least 5 days (Mara & Silva, 1986).

The Engelberg quality guideline for unrestricted irrigation (edible crops, including those eaten raw, sports fields, public parks) comprises the same helminth requirement and a maximum geometric mean concentration of 1000 faecal coliforms per 100 ml. The purpose of this latter recommendation is to protect the health of the consumers of the crops, especially vegetable and salad crops. This concentration represents a major relaxation of earlier standards but is in accord with current standards for bathing water quality; in Europe, for example, this standard is <2000 faecal coliforms per 100 ml (Council of the European Communities, 1976), and it makes little sense to demand a standard for irrigation that is more stringent than that for total body immersion. Recent research (Oragui et al., 1987) has confirmed that at a concentration of <1000 faecal coliforms per 100 ml, which implies a very high removal of faecal coliforms (4–$6\log_{10}$ units or $>99.99\%$), bacterial pathogens will be either absent or present in only negligible numbers (see Table 4.6). Effluents of this quality are readily produced by a series of 4–6 waste stabilization ponds with an overall retention time of 20 days or more at temperatures above 20 °C (see Section 7.2). Effluents of a higher quality (<100 faecal coliforms per 100 ml, for example) may be required for wastewater used to irrigate public parks and hotel lawns to protect the health of those, especially tourists and young children, who come into contact with recently irrigated grass.

Box 4.2 Rationale for the Engelberg guidelines for the microbiological quality of treated wastewater used for crop irrigation: the Adelboden statement

The very strict microbial standards developed by the California State Health Department and some other groups some 50 years ago of 2 coliforms per 100 ml for effluent irrigation of vegetables and salad crops eaten uncooked were based on a "zero risk" concept. They were partially motivated by the literature on pathogen detection and survival in wastewater and in soil, which suggested that the mere presence of pathogens in the environment is evidence of a serious public health risk. They may also have been influenced by the public opposition to earlier mismanaged raw sewage farms near residential areas, which aroused public health fears on grounds of odour and fly nuisance. These standards were not really feasible with normal wastewater treatment technologies, even in developed countries, but this was of little concern since the health authorities may well have preferred that unrestricted irrigation did not become a widespread practice. It must also be stated that these strict early standards were not based on an analysis of any epidemiological evidence. The California standard rapidly spread throughout the world to most developing countries as the most commonly accepted guideline for wastewater reuse since no other credible source of evidence on this subject existed. However, for some time experts have questioned the validity of this early approach as being unreasonably strict; for example, a WHO Working Group stated "economically and practically a 'no-risk' level cannot be obtained, although it may be technologically possible" (WHO, 1981).

The participants at the Engelberg meeting critically evaluated the massive amount of epidemiological data reviewed and analysed by the World Bank study (Shuval et al., 1986) and the IRCWD/WHO study (Blum & Feachem, 1985) on credible health effects associated with wastewater and excreta use in agriculture. They unanimously concluded that the risks of irrigation with well treated wastewater were minimal and that current bacterial standards were unjustifiably restrictive. However, they did recognize that in many developing countries the main risks were associated with helminthic diseases and that the safe use of wastewater would require a high degree of helminth removal. Thus, the Engelberg guidelines represent a new, stricter approach concerning the need to reduce helminth egg levels in effluents to 1 or less per litre. This represents a requirement to achieve a very effective helminth removal of some 99.9% by appro-

(Box 4.2 continued)

priate treatment processes. Stabilization ponds are particularly effective in achieving this goal but other technologies are also available. While the Engelberg guidelines do not refer specifically to protozoa of public health importance, such as *Amoeba* and *Giardia*, it was understood that the strict helminth standard recommended was selected as an indicator for all of the large easily settleable pathogens including the protozoa. It is thus implied in the Engelberg guidelines that equally high removals of all protozoa will be achieved.

On the other hand, the Engelberg meeting participants concurred that a microbial standard of some 1000 faecal coliforms per 100 ml for unrestricted crop irrigation was both epidemiologically sound and technologically feasible. They also considered that it was much in line with the actual river water quality used for unrestricted irrigation in Europe and the United States with no known ill effects. The group also noted that many countries found levels of 1000 coliforms per 100 ml acceptable for bathing water quality. It was not considered rational to require a stricter standard for unrestricted irrigation than was considered acceptable for general irrigation and bathing by most of the industrialized countries.

Further, the Engelberg meeting participants felt strongly that the irrational application of unjustifiably strict microbial standards for wastewater irrigation had led to an anomalous situation. Standards were often not enforced at all and serious public health problems resulted from totally unregulated illegal irrigation of salad crops with raw wastewater as is in fact widely practised in many developing countries. The Engelberg approach called for realistic revised standards which were stricter for helminth removal but more feasible regarding bacterial levels. It was the combined epidemiological and engineering judgement of the Engelberg group that this new approach would increase public health protection for a greater number of people with goals which were technologically and economically feasible.

For a full analysis of the epidemiological foundations upon which the Engelberg guidelines are based, the reader is referred to the original reports of Shuval et al. (1986) and Blum & Feachem (1985). These guidelines are intended to guide design engineers in the choice of treatment and management technologies that will reliably achieve the standard. Once achieved, there will be no necessity for the continuous monitoring of indicator organism concentrations.

Table 4.6 Geometric mean bacterial and viral numbers[a] and percentage removals in raw wastewater (RW) and the effluents of five waste stabilization ponds in series (P1–P5)[b] in northeast Brazil at a mean mid-depth pond temperature of 26 °C

Organism	RW	P1	P2	P3	P4	P5	Percentage removal
Faecal coliforms	2×10^7	4×10^6	8×10^5	2×10^5	3×10^4	7×10^3	99.97
Faecal streptococci	3×10^6	9×10^5	1×10^5	1×10^4	2×10^3	300	99.99
Clostridium perfringens	5×10^4	2×10^4	6×10^3	2×10^3	1×10^3	300	99.40
Total bifidobacteria	1×10^7	3×10^6	5×10^4	100	0	0	100.00
Sorbitol-positive bifids	2×10^6	5×10^5	2×10^3	40	0	0	100.00
Campylobacters	70	20	0.2	0	0	0	100.00
Salmonellae	20	8	0.1	0.02	0.01	0	100.00
Enteroviruses	1×10^4	6×10^3	1×10^3	400	50	9	99.91
Rotaviruses	800	200	70	30	10	3	99.63

[a] Bacterial numbers per 100 ml, viral numbers per 10 litres.

[b] P1 was an anaerobic pond with a mean hydraulic retention time of 1 day; P2 and P3–P5 were secondary facultative and maturation ponds respectively, each with a retention time of 5 days. Pond depths were 3.4–2.8 m.

Source: Oragui et al. (1987)

4.4.2 Excreta quality for agricultural use

If excreta and excreta-derived products (such as wastewater sludges, composts, septage and latrine contents) are applied to the field before the planting of crops, no quality guidelines are necessary provided that:

- the wastes are placed in trenches and covered with at least 25 cm of soil;

- farm and sanitation workers are adequately protected during this process; and

- root crops are not planted directly over the trenches.

If the waste products are not buried in trenches but are applied as a topsoil dressing (as is common with composts, for instance), or if they are regularly applied to the soil after planting has occurred (as is usually the case with liquid nightsoil), the Engelberg guidelines for wastewater irrigation should be observed (and interpreted as <1 egg per litre or kilogram (wet weight) and <1000 faecal coliforms per 100 ml or 100 g (wet weight) as appropriate). Treatment of nightsoil to achieve the helminth standard for restricted use can be achieved by various technologies, and composting is an effective way to achieve the standard of <1000 faecal coliforms per 100 g for unrestricted use (see Section 7.2.3).

4.4.3 Excreta and wastewater quality for aquacultural use

Strauss (1985) has reviewed the literature on the survival of pathogens in and on fish. His principal findings were as follows:

- Invasion of fish muscle by bacterial pathogens is very likely to occur when the fish are raised in ponds that contain concentrations of faecal coliforms and salmonellae of $>10^4$ and $>10^5$ per 100 ml respectively; the potential for muscle invasion increases with duration of exposure of the fish to the contaminated water.
- Even at lower contamination levels, high pathogen concentrations may be present in the digestive tract and the intraperitoneal fluid of the fish.

Further work is needed before a definitive bacteriological quality standard can be established for pisciculture, but a tentative interim guideline would be that fish-pond water should contain < 1000 faecal coliforms per 100 ml. The same faecal coliform standard should be applied to ponds in which macrophytes are grown, as these are frequently eaten raw. A further necessary public health measure is to ensure high standards of hygiene during fish handling and especially gutting. This is more feasible in the case of commercial operations than in the case of subsistence aquaculture, for which sustained health education programmes will often be required.

The transmission of clonorchiasis and fasciolopsiasis occurs only in very restricted geographical areas of Asia (see Figures 4.7 and 4.8). Given the cultural preference in these areas for eating raw fish and aquatic vegetables — the second intermediate hosts of these pathogens — transmission can be prevented only by ensuring that no eggs enter the pond or by snail control. The latter option is unlikely to be

Figure 4.7 Known geographical distribution of *Clonorchis sinensis*

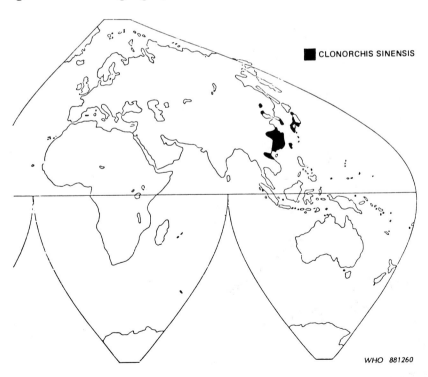

■ CLONORCHIS SINENSIS

WHO 881260

From Feachem et al. (1983), reproduced by permission of the World Bank

Figure 4.8 Known geographical distribution *of Fasciolopsis buski*

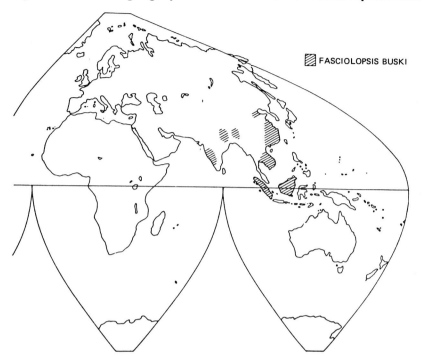

From Feachem et al. (1983), reproduced by permission of the World Bank

continuously achieved in practice, especially in the small subsistence ponds common in parts of Asia. Thus the only feasible means of control is to remove all viable trematode eggs before excreta and wastewater are applied to ponds — *all* eggs must be rendered non-viable because of the huge asexual multiplication of the pathogen in its first intermediate host. Similar considerations apply to the control of schistosomiasis, which is a potential occupational risk to both fish- and macrophyte-pond workers in a much wider geographical area (see Figures 4.9 and 4.10). The appropriate helminthic quality guideline for all aquacultural use of excreta and wastewater is thus the absence of viable trematode eggs. This is readily achieved in wastewater by pond treatment and in excreta by storage for at least one month (see Section 7.2.4).

Tentative microbiological quality guidelines for aquacultural use, analogous to the Engelberg guidelines for agricultural use, are given in Table 4.7.

Figure 4.9 Known geographical distribution of *Schistosoma haematobium, S. japonicum* and *S. mekongi*

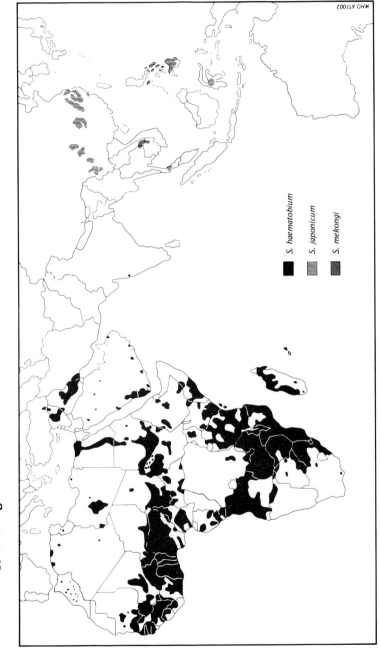

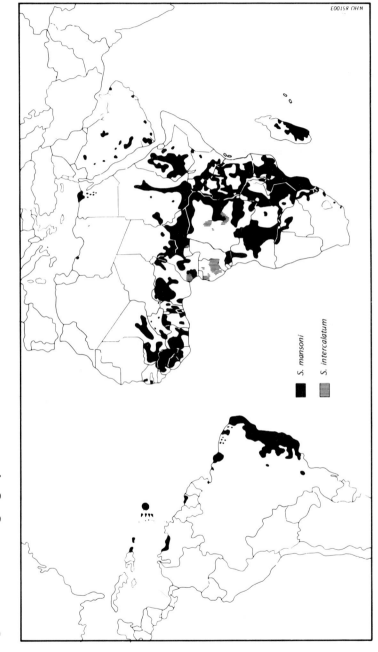

Figure 4.10 Known geographical distribution of *Schistosoma mansoni* and *S. intercalatum*

S. mansoni

S. intercalatum

Table 4.7 Tentative microbiological quality criteria for the aquacultural use of wastewater and excreta

Reuse process	Viable trematode eggs[a] (arithmetic mean number per litre or kg)	Faecal coliforms (geometric mean number per 100 ml or per 100 g)[b]
Fish culture	0	$< 10^4$
Aquatic macrophyte culture	0	$< 10^4$

[a] *Clonorchis, Fasciolopsis* and *Schistosoma*. Consideration need be given to this guideline only in endemic areas (Figures 4.7–4.10).
[b] This guideline assumes that there is a one $\log_{10}$ unit reduction in faecal coliforms occurring in the pond, so that in-pond concentrations are < 1000 per 100 ml. If consideration of pond temperature and retention time indicates that a higher reduction can be achieved, the guideline may be relaxed accordingly.

5
Sociocultural aspects

Human behavioural patterns are a key determining factor in the transmission of excreta-related diseases. The social feasibility of changing certain behavioural patterns in order to introduce excreta or wastewater use schemes, or to reduce disease transmission in existing schemes, can be assessed only with a prior understanding of the cultural values attached to practices that appear to be social preferences yet which facilitate disease transmission. Cultural beliefs vary so widely in different parts of the world that it is not possible to assume that any of the practices that have evolved in relation to excreta and wastewater use (see Table 2.1, page 24) can be readily transferred elsewhere: a thorough assessment of the local sociocultural context is always necessary (Cross, 1985).

5.1 Excreta use

Human society has evolved very different sociocultural responses to the use of untreated excreta, ranging from abhorrence through disaffection and indifference to predilection. For example, in Africa, the Americas and Europe, excreta use is generally regarded with disaffection or, at best, indifference. This results from the strongly held view that human excreta, especially faeces, are repugnant substances best kept away from the senses of sight and smell. Products fertilized with raw excreta are regarded as tainted or defiled in some way. Such views are not held, or at least not so rigidly, in relation to excreta-derived composts or wastewater sludges, and these materials are commonly used in agriculture, horticulture and land reclamation schemes.

In contrast, both human and animal wastes have been used in agriculture and aquaculture in, for example, China, Japan and Java for thousands of years (see Section 2.3). This practice is in social accord with the Japanese and Chinese traditions of frugality and reflects a deep ecological, as well as economic, appreciation of the dependent relationship between soil fertility and human wastes. In such societies intensive cultivation practices have evolved in response to the need to feed a large number of people living in an area of limited land availability, and this has necessitated the careful use of all the resources available to the community, including excreta. Thus excreta use is dictated by survival economics. Even so, any attempts to minimize health risks by altering the established excreta use practices are likely to meet with social acceptance and success only if the changes are minor and socially unimportant. Any attempts to alter a social preference are likely to fail. Thus excreta storage to inactivate trematode eggs is likely to be a feasible change to the belief that fresh (i.e. untreated) excreta must be used for maximal agricultural benefit, but exhortations not to eat raw fish are likely to fall on deaf ears.

In Islamic societies direct contact with excreta is abhorred, since by Koranic edict it is regarded as containing impurities (*najassa*). Its use is permitted only when the *najassa* have been removed. Thus the agricultural use of untreated excreta would not be tolerated, and any attempt to modify this would be futile. On the other hand, excreta use after treatment would be acceptable if the treatment is such that the *najassa* are removed — for example, after thermophilic composting which produces a humus-like substance that has no visual or odorous connection with the original material. *Najassa* may be deemed to be removed in other ways. In Java, for example, it is acceptable to fertilize fish-ponds with untreated excreta because the excreta are diluted by the pond water and because the water flows from one pond to the next; this combination of dilution and flow is considered to render the water pure (*tahur*), and so the practice is religiously acceptable.

In many developing countries the task of collecting urban nightsoil is regarded as employment of very low status, and consequently it is becoming increasingly difficult for urban authorities to recruit people for such work. As a result, sanitation facilities that produce nightsoil, such as bucket latrines, are being replaced by those that do not, for example pour-flush latrines. Indeed in some countries, for example India, the government is promoting programmes to replace bucket latrines with pour-flush toilets not only for reasons of improved health but also because of "society's demand for doing away with the degrading practice of human beings carrying nightsoil loads" (Venugopalan, 1984). There is therefore a trend for nightsoil to be replaced by latrine sludges as the raw material in excreta use schemes. From the viewpoint of excreta-related disease control this is to be welcomed as the pathogen load, and hence the potential risk to health, is substantially reduced.

5.2 Wastewater use

Untreated wastewater is currently used for crop irrigation in many parts of the world where it is produced, and there does not appear to be any significant sociocultural revulsion at this practice. (This is not always the case, however, and the practice may be initiated only by economic necessity.) Treated wastewater is much less objectionable in appearance than untreated wastewater and from a socio-aesthetic viewpoint is more suitable for agricultural and aquacultural use. Any public fears may be allayed by suitably designed information programmes.

In Islamic countries wastewater may be used for irrigation provided that the impurities (*najassa*) present in raw wastewater are removed. Untreated wastewater is in fact used in some Islamic countries, principally in areas where there is an extreme water shortage and then generally from a local wadi (ephemeral desert stream), but this is clearly a result of economic need and not of cultural preference. According to Farooq & Ansari (1983) there are three ways in which impure water may be transformed into pure water:

- self-purification of the water (for example, removal of the impurities by sedimentation);

- addition of pure water in sufficient quantity to dilute the impurities; and

- removal of the impurities by the passage of time or physical effects (for example, sunlight and wind).

It is notable that the first and third of these transformations are essentially similar to those achieved by modern wastewater treatment processes, especially stabilization ponds.

6
Environmental aspects

Excreta and wastewater use schemes, if properly planned and managed, can have a positive environmental impact as well as increasing agricultural and aquacultural yields. Environmental improvement occurs as a result of several factors, the most important of which are the following:

- Avoidance of surface water pollution, which would occur if the wastewater were not used but discharged into rivers or lakes. Major environmental pollution problems, such as depletion of dissolved oxygen, eutrophication, foaming and fish kills, can be avoided.

- Conservation or more rational use of freshwater resources, especially in arid and semi-arid areas; fresh water for urban demand, wastewater for agricultural use.

- Reduced requirements for artificial fertilizers, with a concomitant reduction in energy expenditure and industrial pollution elsewhere.

- Soil conservation through humus build-up and through the prevention of land erosion.

- Desertification control and desert reclamation, through irrigation and fertilization of tree belts.

- Improved urban amenities, through irrigation and fertilization of green spaces for recreation (parks, sports facilities) and visual appeal (flowers, shrubs and trees adjacent to urban roads and highways).

Pollution of soil and ground water is clearly a potential disadvantage of using excreta and wastewater in agriculture. Under most conditions, wastewater irrigation does not present a microbiological threat to ground water since it is a process similar to slow sand filtration: most of the pathogens are retained in the top few metres of the soil, and horizontal travel distances in uniform soil conditions are normally less than 20 m. However, in certain hydro-geological situations (for example, in limestone formations) microbial pollutants can be transported for much greater distances, and careful investigation is required in such cases (see Lewis et al., 1982). Chemical pollutants, among which nitrates are of principal concern in the case of domestic wastes, can travel for greater distances, and there is the potential risk that drinking-water supplies in the vicinity of wastewater irrigation projects may be affected. Generally, water supplies should not be located within, or close to, wastewater-irrigated fields.

As a result of increased rates of salinization and waterlogging, soil pollution can occur through wastewater irrigation if inadequate attention is paid to leaching and drainage requirements. Saline drainage waters should be used to irrigate salt-tolerant crops where possible, and crop and field rotation will generally be necessary to avoid long-term damage to the soil structure. Adherence to good irrigation practice is essential to avoid adverse environmental effects, and standard texts should be consulted for further details (for example, Rydzewski, 1987; Pettygrove & Asano, 1984; Ayers & Westcot, 1985). Often a trade-off has to be made between agricultural production and environmental protection, and this must be carefully evaluated at the project planning stage (see Section 8). Many of the above potential disadvantages of wastewater irrigation, together with such hazards as odour, vector development and the effects of accidental discharges of toxic substances, can be avoided by the use of properly treated wastewater (see Section 7).

Excreta use in agriculture and aquaculture has many of the advantages of wastewater use, and fewer potential environmental disadvantages. Most on-site sanitation systems can be easily de-signed or adapted for reuse, and the resulting latrine sludges can be safely used. The production of excreta-derived compost by using pulverized domestic refuse to correct the carbon-to-nitrogen ratio and moisture content of excreta (see Section 7.2.3) has the greatest potential for environmental improvement, through the reclamation and subsequent use of the two worst visual pollutants of the urban environment in developing countries — excreta and domestic refuse. Excreta-derived compost is a valuable, pathogen-free soil conditioner and fertilizer. Its production and use provide a simple and environmentally advantageous solution to both human wastes reuse and environmental pollution in urban areas without a sewerage system.

7
Technical options for health protection

7.1 Introduction

The single most effective and reliable strategy for preventing transmission of disease caused by the use of human wastes is to treat the wastes according to the Engelberg quality guidelines (see Section 4.4). If this is done, disease transmission to those working in or living near the fields or ponds, and also to the crop-consuming public, either ceases or is reduced to a level of epidemiological insignificance.

However, such thorough treatment may be expensive or unfeasible or may even be unnecessary since the presence of human pathogens in fields or ponds need not represent a health risk if other suitable health protection measures are taken. These measures may prevent pathogens from reaching the worker or the crop or, by selection of appropriate crops (cotton for example), may prevent any pathogens on the crop from affecting the consumer. The available measures for health protection can thus be grouped under four main headings:

- treatment of the waste;

- crop restriction;

- waste application methods;

- control of human exposure.

The points at which these measures can interrupt the potential routes of transmission of excreted pathogens are illustrated in Figure 7.1.

It will often be desirable to apply a combination of several methods. For example, crop restriction may be sufficient to protect consumers but will need to be supplemented by additional measures to protect agricultural workers. Sometimes, partial treatment to a less demanding standard may be sufficient if combined with other

Figure 7.1 Effect of health protection measures in interrupting potential transmission routes of excreted pathogens

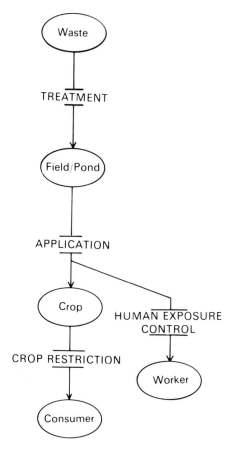

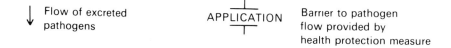

| ↓ Flow of excreted pathogens | APPLICATION | Barrier to pathogen flow provided by health protection measure |

measures. The concept is illustrated in a schematic and simplified way in Figure 7.2, which shows three combinations that can success-fully protect the health of both workers and consumers. The feasibility and efficacy of any combination will depend on many factors, which must be carefully considered before any option is put into practice. These factors will include the following:

- availability of resources (manpower, funds, land);

Figure 7.2 Generalized model to show the level of risk to human health associated with different combinations of control measures for the use of wastewater or excreta in agriculture or aquaculture

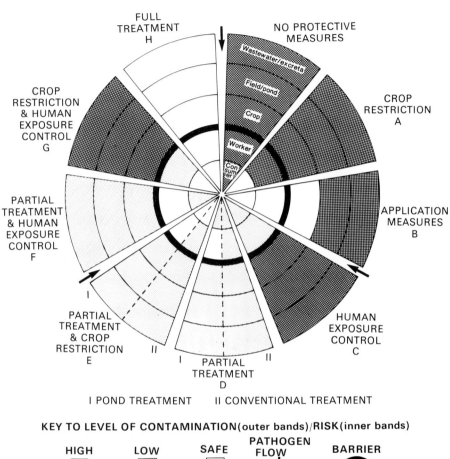

FULL TREATMENT
H

NO PROTECTIVE MEASURES

CROP RESTRICTION & HUMAN EXPOSURE CONTROL
G

CROP RESTRICTION
A

PARTIAL TREATMENT & HUMAN EXPOSURE CONTROL
F

APPLICATION MEASURES
B

PARTIAL TREATMENT & CROP RESTRICTION
E

HUMAN EXPOSURE CONTROL
C

PARTIAL TREATMENT
D

I POND TREATMENT   II CONVENTIONAL TREATMENT

KEY TO LEVEL OF CONTAMINATION(outer bands)/RISK(inner bands)

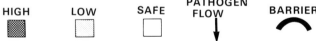

HIGH   LOW   SAFE   PATHOGEN FLOW   BARRIER

- existing social and agricultural practices;

- existing patterns of excreta-related disease.

For example, if funds or land are not available for wastewater treatment to the Engelberg guideline quality for unrestricted irrigation (see Table 4.5, page 79), some of the other three types of health protection measure will be needed. In some cases, suitable crop restriction can make it unnecessary to take any further measures to protect the public. On the other hand, if staff shortages and existing practices make it impossible to implement and enforce crop restrictions effectively, recourse must be made to other methods. In the case of aquacultural use, it will be possible to ignore the guideline for waste quality (see Table 4.7, page 89) if trematode infections are not found in the project area. Small-scale reuse schemes, especially for excreta, require special attention. They are often subsistence-level operations that are difficult to control and in which treatment is generally impossible; measures often need to be developed for minimization of risk to the individual, including health education and improved domestic water supplies.

The technical factors affecting each option are discussed below. Administrative and financial factors, which are equally important, are discussed in Section 8.

7.2 Wastes treatment

7.2.1 Objectives

The objective in treating wastewater or excreta for use in agriculture or aquaculture is to remove excreted pathogens and thus prevent disease transmission. However, this is not the purpose for which conventional wastewater treatment systems, normally used in Europe and North America, were originally developed. Their primary objective was the removal of organic matter, expressed in terms of their biochemical or chemical oxygen demand, and suspended solid material. In recent years, with increasing awareness of environmental pollution, sophisticated tertiary treatment processes have been added to conventional systems to improve pathogen removal. Waste stabilization ponds constitute a much simpler method of pathogen removal.

In considering pathogen removal from wastes, the number of pathogens surviving is more important than the number removed or killed. Figures such as 99% or 99.9% removal may seem very impressive, but they represent 1% or 0.1% survival respectively, and in view of the high concentrations of pathogens that can occur in the wastes, these proportions can be significant. Raw sewage may contain over 10^5 pathogenic bacteria per litre so that 99% removal would still leave over 10^3 pathogenic bacteria per litre.

The degree of removal by a waste treatment process is therefore best expressed in terms of $\log_{10}$ units: 99% removal is equivalent to two log units of reduction. From that perspective, there is only a trivial difference between a process that achieves 92% removal and one that removes 98%. Raw domestic wastewater typically contains about 10^7 faecal coliforms per 100 ml, and some 10^3 helminth eggs per litre where helminth infections are prevalent. To achieve the Engelberg guideline quality for unrestricted irrigation, therefore, a bacterial reduction of at least 4 log units and a helminth egg removal of 3 log units are required.

A lesser degree of removal can be considered if other health protection measures are envisaged or if the quality will be further improved after treatment. This can occur by dilution in naturally occurring water, by prolonged storage or by transport over long distances in a river or canal. The degree of pathogen reduction by dilution is easy to estimate, but the relevant figure to use is the minimum dilution, and this occurs in the dry season when stream flows are at their lowest. Pathogen reduction in reservoirs, rivers and channels is primarily a function of time and temperature and not necessarily of distance downstream. Pathogens in a fast-flowing natural stream may travel 50 km in little more than 12 hours, which is not likely to be sufficient time for any significant reduction in their numbers to occur.

7.2.2 Wastewater treatment

In the present context of wastewater reuse, the removal of excreted pathogens is the principal treatment objective. Efficient removal requires processes specifically designed for this purpose; incidental removal in other processes developed for other purposes is unlikely to be cost-effective (see Box 7.1). The removal of excreted pathogens in wastewater treatment processes has been reviewed in detail by Feachem et al. (1983). Table 7.1 summarizes the available information for the excreted bacteria and helminths and indicates where the Engelberg guidelines can be met. Degrees of removal of viruses and cysts are also given in Table 7.1, although these are not relevant to achievement of the Engelberg guidelines.

Conventional (primary and secondary) treatment

Raw wastewaters contain 10^7–10^9 faecal coliforms per 100 ml and it is clear from Table 7.1 that conventional processes (plain sedimentation, activated sludge, biofiltration, aerated lagoons and oxidation ditches) are not able, unless supplemented by disinfection, to produce an effluent that complies with the Engelberg guideline for bacterial quality (< 1000 faecal coliforms per 100 ml).

Conventional wastewater treatment systems are not generally effective for helminth egg removal. There is a need for research and

Box 7.1 Wastewater treatment costs

A recent World Bank report gives a detailed economic comparison of waste stabilization ponds, aerated lagoons, oxidation ditches and biological filters. The data for this cost comparison were taken from the city of San'a in the Yemen Arab Republic. Certain assumptions were made, for example the use of maturation ponds to follow the aerated lagoon, and the chlorination of the oxidation ditch and biological filter effluents, in order that the four processes would have a similar bacteriological quality so that fish farming and effluent reuse for irrigation were feasible. The design is based on a population of 250 000; a per capita flow and BOD_5 (biochemical oxygen demand measured on day 5 of treatment) contribution of 120 litres/day and 40 g/day respectively; influent and required effluent faecal coliform concentrations of 2×10^7 and 1×10^4 per 100 ml, respectively; and a required effluent BOD_5 of 25 mg/litre. The calculated land area requirements and total net present worth of each system (assuming an opportunity cost of capital of 12% and land values of US$ 5/m^2) are shown in the table below. The waste stabilization pond is the cheapest option. Clearly the preferred solution is very sensitive to the price of land, and the above cost of US$ 5 per m^2 represents a reasonable value for low-cost housing estates in developing countries.

The cost of chlorination accounts for US$ 0.22 million per year of the operational costs of the last two options.

	Waste stabilization pond system	Aerated lagoon system	Oxidation ditch system	Conventional treatment (biofilters)
Costs (million US$)				
Capital	5.68	6.98	4.80	7.77
Operational	0.21	1.28	1.49	0.86
Benefits (million US$)				
Irrigation income	0.43	0.43	0.43	0.43
Pisciculture income	0.30	0.30	–	–
Net present worth (million US$)	5.16	7.53	5.86	8.20
Land area (ha)	46	50	20	25

Source: Arthur (1983).

development work to improve the helminth egg removal efficacy of conventional systems to meet the Engelberg standards. Such processes as lime treatment, chemical coagulation and sedimentation, upward-flow anaerobic sludge blanket, sand filtration and storage in compartmentalized reservoirs deserve further study.

Table 7.1 Expected removal of excreted bacteria and helminths in various wastewater treatment processes

Treatment process	Removal ($\log_{10}$ units)			
	Bacteria	Helminths	Viruses	Cysts
Primary sedimentation				
Plain	0–1	0–2	0–1	0–1
Chemically assisted[a]	1–2	1–3 (E)	0–1	0–1
Activated sludge[b]	0–2	0–2	0–1	0–1
Biofiltration[b]	0–2	0–2	0–1	0–1
Aerated lagoon[c]	1–2	1–3 (E)	1–2	0–1
Oxidation ditch[b]	1–2	0–2	1–2	0–1
Disinfection[d]	2–6 (E)	0–1	0–4	0–3
Waste stabilization ponds[e]	1–6 (E)	1–3 (E)	1–4	1–4
Effluent storage reservoirs[f]	1–6 (E)	1–3 (E)	1–4	1–4

E—With good design and proper operation the Engelberg guidelines are achievable.
[a] Further research is needed to confirm performance
[b] Including secondary sedimentation
[c] Including settling pond
[d] Chlorination, ozonation
[e] Performance depends on number of ponds in series
[f] Performance depends on retention time, which varies with demand

Source: Feachem et al. (1983).

Waste stabilization ponds

Waste stabilization ponds are usually the wastewater treatment method of choice in warm climates wherever land is available at reasonable cost (Mara, 1976; Arthur, 1983). They should be arranged in a series of anaerobic, facultative and maturation ponds with an overall hydraulic retention time of 10–50 days, depending on the design temperature and the effluent quality required. Pond series can be readily designed to produce effluents that meet the Engelberg guidelines for both bacterial and helminthic quality; these effluents are also low in BOD and suspended solids (see Table 7.2).

The degree of bacterial reduction in a pond can be estimated from the formula:

$$R = 1 + Kt$$

where R is the ratio between the concentrations of faecal coliforms in the incoming and outflowing water; t is the retention time of the pond in days (i.e. its volume divided by the flow through it); and K is a factor representing the rate of die-off of faecal bacteria, which

Table 7.2 Performance of a series of five waste stabilization ponds in north-east Brazil (mean pond temperature: 26 °C)

Sample	Retention time (days)	BOD$_5$ (mg/l)	Suspended solids (mg/l)	Faecal coliforms	Intestinal nematode eggs (per litre)
Raw wastewater	–	240	305	4.6×10^7	804
Effluent from:					
Anaerobic pond	6.8	63	56	2.9×10^6	29
Facultative pond	5.5	45	74	3.2×10^5	1
Maturation pond 1	5.5	25	61	2.4×10^4	0
Maturation pond 2	5.5	19	43	450	0
Maturation pond 3	5.8	17	45	30	0

Source: Mara et al. (1983), Mara & Silva (1986).

depends on temperature. For maturation ponds, K can be estimated from:

$$K = 2.6 \ (1.19)^{T-20}$$

where T is the mean temperature in °C. The mean monthly temperature of the coldest month of the year is normally used for design purposes (Mara, 1976). For facultative ponds, bacterial die-off rates are slightly slower. The degree of reduction in a series of ponds can be calculated from the fact that R_s for the series as a whole is simply the product of the values of R for the individual ponds:

$$R_s = R_1 \cdot R_2 \cdot R_3 \ldots$$

The relationship between temperature, retention time and the reduction ratio R for a single pond is shown in Figure 7.3.

A number of ponds connected together in series will give better pathogen removal than a single pond with the same total retention time. Examples of the effluent quality that has been obtained in several series of ponds are given in Table 7.3. Each of these series had a total retention time of more than 25 days, but in many cases this could be reduced without jeopardizing the achievement of the Engelberg guideline.

Recent research in northeastern Brazil (Mara & Silva, 1986) has shown that the Engelberg guideline for helminths would normally be achieved by a series of three ponds—a 1-day anaerobic pond followed by a 5-day facultative pond and a

**Figure 7.3 Reduction of faecal coliform bacteria in waste stabiliza-
tion ponds as a function of time and removal**

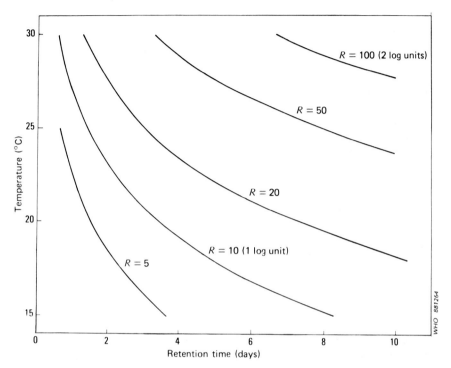

The reduction factor R is the number of faecal coliforms in the pond influent
divided by that in the effluent

**Table 7.3 Reported effluent quality for several series of waste
stabilization ponds, each with a retention time > 25 days**

Pond system	No. of ponds in series	Effluent quality (FC/100 ml)[a]
Australia, Melbourne	8–11	100
Brazil, Campina Grande[b]	5	30
France, Porquerolles	3	100
Jordan, Amman	9	30
Peru, Lima	5	100
Tunisia, Tunis	4	200

[a] FC = Faecal coliforms
[b] Experimental Centre for Biological Treatment of Wastewater (Extrabes).

Source: Bartone & Arlosoroff (1987).

103

5-day maturation pond. Such a series would, depending on temperature, reduce the faecal coliform concentration by only 2–3 $\log_{10}$ units, so that further maturation ponds would be necessary in order to achieve the Engelberg guideline of < 1000 per 100 ml. The size and number of the maturation ponds control the number of faecal coliforms in the final effluent of the pond series, and the design process (see Gambrill et al., 1986) specifically selects the optimum combination of maturation pond size and number required to achieve the desired final effluent quality.

The high degree of confidence with which pond series can be designed to produce effluents meeting the Engelberg guidelines is only one of the many advantages of pond systems. Others are:

- lower costs (for construction, operation and maintenance) than other treatment processes;

- no expenditure of energy (other than solar energy);

- high ability to absorb organic and hydraulic shock loads;

- extreme simplicity of operation and maintenance;

- ability to treat a wide variety of industrial and agricultural wastes.

The only disadvantage of pond systems is the relatively large area of land that they require, and this may limit their use, especially in metropolitan areas. Increasing pond depth is one method of reducing land area requirements, and recent research (Oragui et al., 1987; Mara et al., 1987) has shown that ponds 2–3 m deep can achieve degrees of bacterial and viral removal comparable to those in ponds of conventional depth (1–1.5 m). Further research is needed to determine other ways in which pond land area requirements can be minimized, for example by using ponds in conjunction with other more compact methods of treatment, such as soil/aquifer treatment. However, operation and maintenance requirements will be significantly more complex. In many situations, conventional pond systems are the best method of producing wastewater effluents suitable for crop irrigation.

Tertiary treatment

Tertiary treatment processes were originally developed to improve the quality of secondary (activated sludge or biofilter) effluents, mainly to reduce further the BOD and concentrations of suspended solids or to remove nutrients, although some processes (for example disinfection) were developed to reduce the number of excreted pathogens.

Processes designed to improve physicochemical quality — such as rapid sand filtration, nitrification-denitrification, and carbon adsorption — have little or no effect on excreted bacterial removal, but some of them (for example filtration) may be effective in removing helminths; further research is needed to provide reliable design data. However, these processes are usually complicated and expensive technologies, and their use in developing countries to produce suitable effluents for crop irrigation is unwarranted.

Disinfection

Disinfection — usually chlorination — of raw sewage has never been fully successful in practice. It can be used to reduce the numbers of excreted bacteria in the effluent from a conventional treatment plant if the plant is operating well. A chlorine dose of 10–30 mg/l is usually required, with a contact time of 30–60 minutes. The dose required must be verified by laboratory tests, as it varies widely with the concentration of organic matter in the waste.

However, as stressed by Chambers (1971): "Chlorination of wastewater effluents is a vastly more complex and unpredictable operation than chlorination of water supplies. It is extremely difficult to maintain a high, uniform and predictable level of disinfecting efficiency in any but the most efficiently operated waste treatment plants." For this reason it should not be considered a viable treatment option except where the highest levels of management and process control are guaranteed; irregular or inadequate disinfection is of little use for health protection. In any case, chlorination will leave most helminth eggs totally unharmed, and it is most unlikely that it will be effective in removing protozoal cysts (Feachem et al., 1983).

The environment produced by chlorination of treated effluent, rich in nutrients but low in microbiological activity, is ideal for the growth of some excreted bacteria. Coliforms and other species have been observed to multiply after chlorination to thousands of times the number surviving the initial treatment (Feachem et al., 1983). Effluent chlorination also contributes to the formation and environmental proliferation of chlorinated organic compounds that can be toxic to fish and other aquatic life (Water Research Centre, 1979). However, neither coliform regrowth nor chlorinated organic compounds have yet been reported as significant problems in agricultural use.

A more serious problem is the cost of chlorine — currently about US$ 1.00 per kilogram. Disinfection of the effluent from even a small treatment plant treating only 10 l/s of wastewater with a dose of 30 mg/l will cost about US$ 10 000 each year for the chlorine alone, without counting labour and equipment costs. For many countries, this is a cost in foreign exchange. Other disinfectants such as bromine and ozone may also be used, either alone or together with chlorine. These are usually more expensive still, and not much more effective.

Polishing ponds

A far more appropriate tertiary treatment option is to add one or more ponds in series to a conventional treatment plant. These are essentially the same as the maturation ponds in a series of waste stabilization ponds, and are designed in the same way to give the desired degree of removal of excreted bacteria and helminths. They are particularly suitable for developing countries, as they are reliable and require very little maintenance if they are competently designed and built. The maintenance tasks are simple and more akin to gardening than engineering.

The addition of polishing ponds is a suitable measure to upgrade an existing wastewater treatment plant (see Section 7.2.5).

Storage reservoirs

Demand for irrigation water is usually concentrated in the dry season or in particular periods of the agricultural year, while the flow of wastewater is relatively constant. Large reservoirs, often formed by damming existing watercourses, are therefore often used to store the wastewater until it is needed. Such storage reservoirs are used in Mexico and Israel (Shuval et al., 1986). Further treatment is achieved in such reservoirs, especially with regard to bacterial and helminthic qualities. At present there are insufficient field data on their performance to formulate a rational design process, but it is clear that pathogen removal will be enhanced by dividing them into compartments, connected in series, to reduce the degree of short-circuiting that can occur. The greater the number of compartments, and the longer the minimum retention time, the more efficiently pathogens will be removed.

For an undivided storage reservoir some degree of prior treatment will often be needed. An appropriately conservative design recommendation might be to provide a minimum hydraulic retention time of 10 days during the irrigation season, and to assume only two $\log_{10}$ units reduction of both faecal coliforms and helminth eggs. Thus the effluent being discharged into the reservoir should contain no more than 100 helminth eggs per litre and, if it is to be used for unrestricted irrigation, no more than 100 000 faecal coliforms per 100 ml during the irrigation season.

Physicochemical quality of treated wastewater

The physicochemical quality of treated domestic wastewaters, especially with regard to their electrical conductivity and sodium adsorption ratio (SAR), is normally within the limits for irrigation waters recommended by FAO (see Ayers & Westcot, 1985). Only if the ponds are treating a significant proportion of industrial wastewater is it necessary to check this and also to ensure that the final effluent does not contain harmful concentrations of phytotoxins, especially boron and heavy metals. In cases where treated wastewater has too high an SAR, consideration should be given to reducing it by blending the wastewater with a water (or wastewater) of a lower SAR; in such cases it is generally more appropriate to use the adjusted SAR (Ayers & Westcot, 1985).

Removal of algae from pond effluents is not necessary (in the soil they act as slow-release fertilizers), except where localized irrigation is practised when they may exacerbate problems of clogging of emitters.

7.2.3 Excreta treatment

No treatment is required for excreta or excreta-derived products (such as septage or wastewater sludge) if they are applied to the land by subsurface injection, or placed in trenches before the start of the growing season, as described in Section 4.4.2. For other methods of land application, treatment is required to meet the Engelberg quality guidelines.

To achieve the guideline for helminthic quality (< 1 viable intestinal nematode egg per 100 g), the excreta to be treated must be stored for a period of at least a year at ambient temperatures (see Figure 7.4). This period of storage refers to the whole time interval between excretion and land application, and so includes any time spent in a latrine pit, for example, or in a treatment process such as an

Figure 7.4 Influence of time and temperature on selected bacterial and helminthic pathogens in excreta and sludges

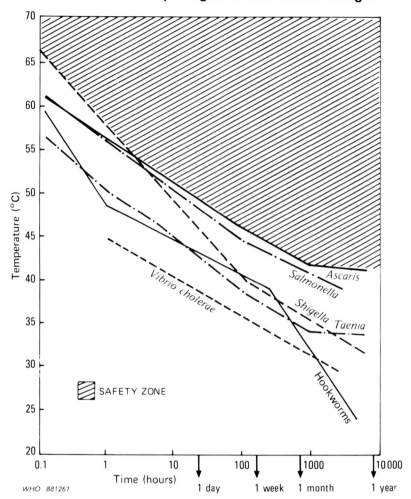

The lines represent conservative upper boundaries for pathogen death — this is, estimates of the time-temperature combinations required for pathogen inactivation. A treatment process with time-temperature effects falling within the zone of safety should be lethal to all excreted bacteria and helminths

From Feachem et al. (1983), reproduced by permission of the World Bank

anaerobic digester or a composting plant. This storage period may be reduced by treatment at a higher temperature, for instance in aerobic composting.

The contents of alternating twin-pit latrines (both ventilated improved pit latrines and pour-flush toilets) require no further treatment after removal from the pit before application to the land, provided that the latrine pits are emptied no more than once a year. Some types of double-pit latrine, such as those used in Guatemala and Viet Nam Guatemala, are normally emptied less than one year after they are filled and sealed. To ensure that the Engelberg guideline is met, the wastes would have to be stored for a further period to ensure that all the waste is at least one year old before use. *All* the contents of single-pit latrines, septic tanks, single-vault compost toilets and wastewater sludges must be stored after removal for at least a year, since there is no way of differentiating between freshly added excreta and that already digested.

Liquid nightsoil (faeces and urine, often with small quantities of toilet flush water) can be simply treated to meet the guidelines for helminthic quality by settlement. Conventional primary sedimentation is not appropriate, however, because of the high solids flux, and a more suitable method is storage for one week, after which the supernatant can be applied to the field. During this storage period, almost all the helminth eggs will settle, thereby posing little health risk to the farm workers who handle the supernatant. The one-week storage time can be readily assured if three storage tanks are available and used in a controlled sequence — one being filled, one undergoing quiescent settling and one in use. The sludge that settles to the bottom of the tank will be very rich in helminth eggs and should be considered in the same way as raw excreta and stored for a minimum period of one year or treated at high temperature. As none of this sludge should be applied directly to the field, simple methods to ensure this should be incorporated in the design of the storage tanks (for example, the installation of a grid just above the maximum sludge level).

Anaerobic mesophilic digestion followed by activated sludge or waste stabilization ponds is commonly used in Japan for treatment of nightsoil, although aerobic thermophilic digestion before activated sludge treatment is becoming more common. However, these are expensive, energy-intensive processes requiring careful operation and maintenance, and they are not generally appropriate in developing countries. A simpler alternative is the direct treatment of nightsoil and septage in waste stabilization ponds.

Elevated-temperature treatment of excreta

Two methods of treating excreta at high temperatures may be used to reduce the minimum storage period of 12 months. These methods will also ensure the removal of faecal coliforms, as well as of helminths, to the Engelberg standard:

(a) **Batch thermophilic digestion** at 50 °C for 13 days will ensure the inactivation of all pathogens. Batch digestion is required to avoid pathogen "shortcircuiting" — which is the term applied when detention times in reactors are lower than is necessary for pathogen inactivation.

(b) **Forced aeration composting:** co-composting of excreta with domestic refuse in aerated static piles (see Figure 7.5) for one month will ensure that the temperature rises to 55–60 °C. Further maturation for 2–4 months at ambient temperature will produce a stable, pathogen-free compost suitable for general horticultural and agricultural use. Alternative bulking agents to domestic refuse, such as rice husks and wood chips, may be used, but from an environmental and municipal point of view domestic refuse is often the most suitable. Excreta may be composted without forced aeration (Gotaas, 1956), and this is likely to be the method of choice for small-scale operations, but pathogen destruction may not be as good or as reliable as with forced aeration (see Box 7.2).

Composting of excreta has several additional advantages:

• it avoids the nuisance of odour and flies associated with the storage and application to the land of raw excreta;

• it conserves nutrients;

Figure 7.5 Schematic diagram of forced aeration co-composting in static piles

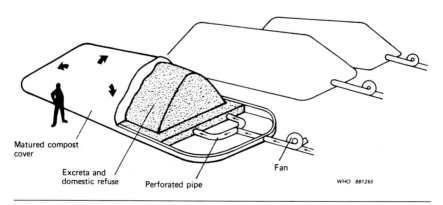

Matured compost cover

Excreta and domestic refuse

Perforated pipe

Fan

WHO 881265

Box 7.2 Forced aeration co-composting of excreta

Excreta (nightsoil) and wastewater sludges do not compost well by themselves: they are too moist and their carbon-to-nitrogen ratio is too low. A co-composting agent, able to absorb the excess moisture and correct the C:N ratio, must be added—for example, refuse, straw, rice husks.

Recent research (Stentiford & Pereira Neto, 1985; Pereira Neto et al., 1986; 1987) has developed the following simple procedure for co-composting:

Aerated pile phase

(a) The materials to be co-composted (20–50 mm in size) are mixed together to give a C:N ratio of 25–35 to 1 with a moisture content of 50–55%.

(b) The static pile is constructed over a length of perforated plastic pipe. Pile dimensions: 1.5–2 m high, 2–4 m wide and 10–50 m long. The pile is covered with an insulating and filtering layer of compost 100 mm thick.

(c) A fan of 250–370 W blows air through the pipe to maintain aerobic conditions within the pile. The fan is operated for 3–5 minutes every 15–20 minutes.

(d) As the temperature rises, the fan acts both to aerate the pile and to maintain a reasonably uniform distribution of temperature. Essentially it pushes heat from the hot inner core to the cooler outer edges, thus avoiding a heat build-up above 60 °C in the central core which would be detrimental to the thermophilic organisms responsible for the composting activity.

(e) The core and edge temperatures are monitored during this thermophilic phase; when they both fall to 35 °C, the pile is dismantled.

Maturation phase

(f) The material from the pile is stored for a further 2–4 months, depending on the ambient temperature, to allow humification of high-carbon compounds, such as lignin and cellulose, to be completed.

After maturation, the compost is screened to remove particles larger than 5–10 mm and it is then ready for agricultural or horticultural use.

- it prevents root damage induced by *in situ* stabilization of organic matter and the resulting free ammonia generation that occurs when raw excreta is applied to the land;

- mature compost helps to control plant pathogens;

- mature compost holds moisture and thus minimizes groundwater pollution, especially by nitrates; and

- soil structure is very much improved, and a fine tilth is easily achieved.

7.2.4 Treatment for aquaculture

Wastewater

For aquatic macrophyte culture, wastewater should be treated to the guideline quality of 0 trematode eggs per litre (see Table 4.7, page 89); this is readily achieved in waste stabilization ponds (see Section 7.2.2). Conventional effluents should be treated in a single polishing (maturation) pond of 5 days' retention time. For fish culture, wastewater should be additionally treated in maturation ponds or by disinfection to a level of less than 1000 faecal coliforms per 100 ml (see Section 4.4.3).

Excreta

Excreta should be treated to the same quality as wastewater. Storage at ambient temperatures renders trematode eggs inviable, and minimum storage periods are as follows:

Clonorchis sinensis	1 week
Fasciolopsis buski	3 weeks
Schistosoma spp	4 weeks

For small-scale operations the triple storage tank method may be used (see Section 7.2.3), but for larger schemes forced aeration composting or batch thermophilic digestion will generally be less expensive.

To achieve the guideline quality of less than 1000 faecal coliforms per 100 ml, excreta should be treated by composting or digestion, or in a series of facultative and maturation ponds with sufficient make-up water being added to replace evaporative losses and ensure an adequate flow through the system.

Pond maintenance

The control of snails, which are the first intermediate host of the trematodes that can be transmitted through aquaculture, can be achieved in fish-ponds by keeping the pond embankments free of vegetation. This vegetation would otherwise provide a suitable shaded habitat for both snails and culicine mosquitos (which may be the local vector of bancroftian filariasis). Such a strategy is not, of course, feasible in the case of macrophyte ponds, for which treatment is the only effective strategy (molluscicide dosing is unfeasible on grounds of cost). Mosquito breeding in macrophyte ponds should be controlled by the introduction of larvivorous fish such as *Gambusia* and *Poecilia*.

7.2.5 Upgrading existing treatment plant

Existing wastewater treatment works may need upgrading to produce an acceptable effluent. The provision of a polishing pond of 5 days' retention time (for helminth egg removal) or additional maturation ponds (for greater removal of faecal coliforms) is an effective solution if sufficient land is available. Alternatively disinfection or chemically assisted secondary sedimentation may be introduced; in the latter case lime or a lime-based coagulant has the advantage over other chemicals of killing faecal bacteria as well as removing helminth eggs, but the effluent pH must be adjusted to below 8.4 by cascade recarbonation or sulfuric acid.

7.3 Crop and fish restriction

7.3.1 Wastewater in agriculture

Wastewater that has been treated to the Engelberg quality guidelines for unrestricted use (< 1000 faecal coliforms per 100 ml and $\leqslant 1$ viable nematode egg per litre) can be used to irrigate any crop, without any further health protection measures. If this standard is not fully met, it may still be possible to grow selected crops without risk to the consumer. Some additional measures will be necessary to protect field workers and crop handlers and may also be required to give full protection to consumers.

Crops can be grouped into three broad categories with regard to the degree to which health protection measures are required (Shuval et al., 1986).

Category A—Protection needed only for field workers

1. Crops not for human consumption (for example cotton, sisal)

2. Crops normally processed by heat or drying before human consumption (grains, oilseeds, sugar-beet)

3. Vegetables and fruit grown exclusively for canning or other processing that effectively destroys pathogens

4. Fodder crops sun-dried and harvested before consumption by animals

5. Landscape irrigation in fenced areas without public access (nurseries, forests, green belts).

Category B—Further measures may be needed

1. Pasture, green fodder crops

2. Crops for human consumption that do not come into direct contact with wastewater, on condition that none must be picked off the ground and that spray irrigation must not be used (tree crops, vineyards, etc.)

3. Crops for human consumption normally eaten only after cooking (potatoes, eggplant, beetroot).

4. Crops for human consumption, the peel of which is not eaten (melons, citrus fruits, bananas, nuts, groundnuts)

5. Any crop if sprinkler irrigation is used (see Section 7.4.1).

Category C—Treatment to Engelberg "unrestricted" guidelines is essential

1. Any crops often eaten uncooked and grown in close contact with wastewater effluent (fresh vegetables such as lettuce or carrots, or spray-irrigated fruit)

2. Landscape irrigation with public access (parks, lawns, golf courses)

Irrigation that is limited to only certain crops and conditions, such as

Category A, is commonly referred to as restricted irrigation.

Crop restriction is a strategy for protection of the consuming public. It has the advantage of providing protection for population groups with lower resistance to infection, including those not part of the indigenous population such as tourists or pilgrims. However, it does not provide protection to the farm workers and their families where a low quality effluent is used in irrigation. Crop restriction is therefore not an adequate single control measure but should be considered within an integrated system of control. To provide protection for the workers as well as for the consumers, it should be complemented by other measures such as partial waste treatment, controlled application of the wastes, or human exposure control (see Figure 7.2).

Compliance only with the helminthic part of the Engelberg quality guideline would be a degree of partial treatment sufficient to protect field workers in most settings and would be cheaper than full treatment. For example, a pond system designed to meet only the helminthic guideline would require 52–67% of the land needed for one designed to reach the faecal coliform guideline, at temperatures of 20–25 °C.

Crop restriction is feasible and is facilitated in several circumstances, including the following:

- where a law-abiding society or strong law enforcement exists;

- where a public body controls allocation of the wastes, and has the legal authority to require that crop restrictions be followed;

- where an irrigation project has strong central management;

- where there is adequate demand for the crops allowed under crop restriction, and where they fetch a reasonable price;

- where there is little market pressure in favour of excluded crops (such as those in Category C).

However, where these circumstances do not prevail, crop restriction programmes will be difficult to enforce. Problems of implementing crop restrictions are further discussed in Section 8.

7.3.2 Excreta in agriculture

As in the case of wastewater irrigation, the restriction of excreta fertilization to Category A crops is a valid strategy for eliminating the health risks to consumers. Risks to field workers and crop handlers can be essentially eliminated by treating the excreta to the Engelberg helminthic quality or by applying it to the land in a suitable way (see Section 7.4.2). If excreta fertilization is used for Category C crops, treatment to the full Engelberg quality guideline is required. If this is not possible, water of a lower quality (but with not more than 10 000 faecal coliforms per 100 ml) may be used to fertilize Category B crops, provided that precautions are taken to control human exposure (see Section 7.5.1).

7.3.3 Aquaculture

Minimization of health risks through crop restriction is not as straightforward in the case of aquacultural use of excreta and wastewater as it is for agricultural use. Most cultured aquatic macrophytes and some fish are sometimes eaten raw in various parts of the world, notably parts of Asia, so that the agricultural option of not using excreta or wastewater for food crops, or for those consumed raw, is often not feasible—it would effectively mean the cessation of traditional aquacultural practices. The introduction of fish that are not eaten raw (for example tilapia) to such areas is a possible solution, but even so it is likely to be difficult to prevent customary practices completely, especially in small-scale subsistence aquaculture.

One practice that appears to be very promising is that of growing "trash" fish, such as tilapia, in excreta- or wastewater-fertilized ponds and feeding them to high-value fish (such as catfish, snakeheads) or crustaceans (shrimps, crayfish) that are reared in freshwater ponds. Insufficient research has been done to determine how contaminated the waste-reared fish may be without contaminating the freshwater-reared fish or crustaceans, but a conservative recommendation would be to grow the trash fish in ponds in which the faecal coliform count is no more than one order of magnitude greater than the guideline value given in Table 4.7 (that is < 10 000 per 100 ml).

7.4 Application of wastewater and excreta

7.4.1 Wastewater in agriculture

Irrigation water, including treated wastewater, can be applied to the land in the five following general ways:

- by flooding (border irrigation), thus wetting almost all the land surface;

- by furrows, thus wetting only part of the ground surface;

- by sprinklers, in which the soil is wetted in much the same way as by rain;

- by subsurface irrigation, in which the surface is wetted little, if at all, but the subsoil is saturated; and

- by localized (trickle, drip or bubbler) irrigation, in which water is applied to each individual plant at an adjustable rate.

The general advantages and disadvantages of these irrigation methods and their suitability for different crops and ground slope conditions are fully discussed in an FAO paper (Doneen & Westcot, 1984), which should be consulted for further details. In specific relation to disease transmission control, the five methods of wastewater application have the advantages and disadvantages listed in Table 7.4. If the treated wastewater is of Engelberg guideline

Table 7.4 Factors affecting choice of irrigation method, and special measures required when wastewater is used

Irrigation method	Factors affecting choice	Special measures for wastewater
Border (flooding) irrigation	Lowest cost, exact levelling not required	Thorough protection for field workers, crop-handlers and consumers
Furrow irrigation	Low cost, levelling may be needed	Protection for field workers, possibly for crop-handlers and consumers
Sprinkler irrigation	Medium water use efficiency, levelling not required	Some Category B crops, especially tree fruit, should not be grown. Minimum distance 50–100 m from houses and roads. Anaerobic wastes should not be used because of odour nuisance
Subsurface and localized irrigation	High cost, high water use efficiency, higher yields	Filtration to prevent clogging of emitters.

quality, any of the five methods may be safely used, the choice between them being based on cost, water availability and ground slope.

If the water is not of this quality, but it is desired to use it on crops in Category B (see Section 7.3.1), sprinkler irrigation should not be used except for pasture or fodder crops, and border irrigation should not be used for vegetables.

Subsurface or localized irrigation can give the greatest degree of health protection as well as using water more efficiently and often producing higher yields (see Box 7.3). However, it is expensive and has not yet been used on a wide scale for irrigation with wastewater. A high degree of reliable treatment (usually involving both deep-bed and in-line filtration) is required to prevent clogging of the small holes (emitters) through which water is slowly released into the soil.

Bubbler irrigation, a technique developed for localized irrigation of tree crops (see Hillel, 1987), avoids the need for small emitter apertures to regulate the flow to each tree. A 6 mm diameter vertical riser tube is connected to the pipeline, through which water is distributed at low pressure. Each riser tube is supported if necessary by a small stake, and the top is cut off at a carefully chosen level to ensure an equal flow of water "bubbling" (or dribbling) from each tube, irrespective of variations in the ground level. The water runs into a small depression dug around each tree or bush.

If wastewater of lower quality is used, it is essential to follow the recommendations given in Section 7.5.1 for human exposure control in addition to the above restrictions.

Box 7.3 Trickle irrigation of cotton with pond effluent

A trickle system was installed in a cotton field to study the effects of pond effluent quality, emitter discharge and irrigation regime on the yield of cotton. The experiments were conducted in a typical arid zone (Beer-Sheva Valley, Israel) and the cotton was grown on loess soil. The results show that a high cotton yield of more than 6000 kg/ha can be obtained with the use of a high frequency (every 2 days) trickle irrigation system. A total of approximately 5900 m^3 of effluent per hectare was applied, with no additional fertilization required. With proper screen filtration no emitter clogging was observed.

Source: Oron et al. (1982).

7.4.2 Excreta in agriculture

Untreated or insufficiently treated excreta should only be applied to land by placing it in covered trenches before the start of the growing season (see Section 4.4.2), or by subsurface injection using specialized equipment (see Water Research Centre, 1984). Properly composted excreta can be manually or mechanically spread on land without any health risk as it is a pathogen-free material. Settled or thermophilically digested nightsoil may be applied either manually (by bucket and dipper, for example, as is common in China) or by tanker (which is often animal-drawn). The nightsoil, if treated only to the Engelberg guideline for helminthic quality, may contain high concentrations of bacterial and viral pathogens, and these will pose a greater risk to field workers than is the case for restricted irrigation with wastewater, which can only be minimized by exposure control.

7.4.3 Aquaculture

Before marketing, shellfish are commonly held in clean water to remove excreted organisms—a process known as depuration. Depuration is often recommended in excreta-fed aquaculture systems and can be carried out either by stopping application of the waste or by removing the fish to clean ponds. Keeping fish in clean water for at least 2 to 3 weeks before harvest will remove any residual objectionable odours and reduce the degree of contamination with faecal microorganisms. However, such depuration does not guarantee complete removal of pathogens from fish tissues and digestive tracts, unless the contamination is very slight.

7.5 Human exposure control

7.5.1 Agriculture

Four groups of people can be identified as being at potential risk from the agricultural use of wastewater and excreta. These are:

- agricultural field workers and their families;

- crop-handlers;

- consumers (of crops, meat and milk);

- those living near the affected fields.

Agricultural field workers are at high potential risk, especially of parasitic infections (see Section 4.3). Exposure to hookworm infection can be reduced, and even eliminated, by the continuous in-field use of appropriate footwear, but persuading workers to adopt this precaution may be difficult. A rigorous health education programme is needed. A similar approach may be taken with crop-handlers; the risk to them is somewhat less than that to field workers, but it can be reduced by meticulous personal hygiene and the wearing of gloves.

Immunization is not feasible against helminthic infections or against most diarrhoeal diseases. However, for highly exposed groups, immunization against typhoid and administration of immunoglobulin to protect against hepatitis A may be worth considering.

Additional protection may be provided by the availability of adequate medical facilities to treat diarrhoeal disease, and by regular chemotherapy. This might include chemotherapeutic control of intense nematode infections in children and control of anaemia. Chemotherapy must be reapplied at regular intervals to be effective. The frequency required to keep worm burdens at a low level (for example, as low as in the rest of the population) depends on the intensity of transmission, but will not normally be less than once a year. The drugs involved normally cost about US$ 0.50 for each complete treatment. One to three doses are required, depending on which drug is used.

Chemotherapy and immunization cannot normally be considered as an adequate strategy to protect farm workers and their families who are exposed to raw wastewater or excreta. However, where such workers are organized within structured situations such as government or company farms, these could be beneficial as palliative measures, pending improvement in the quality of the wastes used.

Risks to consumers can be reduced by the thorough cooking of vegetables and meat, by boiling milk, and by maintaining high standards of personal and kitchen hygiene. Food hygiene should be included in health education campaigns, although the efficacy of such campaigns may often be quite low in poorly educated societies or outside institutional settings.

Any risk of tapeworm transmission can be controlled by meat inspection provided that animals are slaughtered only in recognized abattoirs where all carcasses are inspected and all infected carcasses are rejected. Although *Taenia* eggs have been known to survive for several months on grazing land, the risk of bovine cysticercosis may be reduced by ceasing the application of the wastes at least two weeks before cattle are allowed to graze.

Wastewater irrigation of fruit trees should also cease two weeks before the fruit is picked.

Local residents should be kept fully informed about the location of all fields where human wastes are used, so that they may avoid entering them and prevent their children from doing so. Warning notices should be posted along the edges of fields, especially if there are no fences.

There is no epidemiological evidence that those living near wastewater-irrigated fields are at significant risk from pathogens present in aerosols from sprinkler irrigation schemes. However, steps should of course be taken to protect residents from direct wetting by droplets of spray from the sprinklers. For this reason, and allowing a reasonable margin of safety, sprinklers should not be used within 50–100 m of houses or roads. This minimum distance will often have to be increased for other reasons, for instance to minimize odour nuisance.

7.5.2 Aquaculture

There are four groups of people at potential risk from the aquacultural use of excreta and wastewater:

- aquacultural pond workers;

- fish- and macrophyte-handlers;

- fish- and macrophyte-consumers;

- those living near ponds fertilized with excreta or wastewater.

Many people will belong to more than one of these groups and thus be doubly at risk. The pond workers are at high potential risk, especially of parasitic infections.

Schistosomiasis is best dealt with by treatment of infected persons and by snail control (see Section 7.2.4). Where this is not possible, exposure to schistosomiasis can be controlled by the wearing of wellington boots or high-body waders (depending on the depth of the pond), but their use is rare and would interfere, for example, with the practice of harvesting lotus by loosening their roots with the toes. When all else fails, regular chemotherapy would be beneficial in endemic areas.

Local residents should be informed which ponds are fertilized with excreta or wastewater, so that they may prevent their children from playing or swimming in them. Warning notices should be posted by ponds adjacent to roads, especially if they are unfenced. However, where there is no adequate water supply or sanitation, local residents are likely to continue using the pond water for bathing, defecation and other purposes. Water supply and sanitation are therefore important measures for human exposure control.

Produce-handlers are at much less risk, and their exposure can be controlled by the wearing of gloves and the adoption of a high level of personal hygiene.

Attempts to alter traditional preferences for consuming aquacultural produce raw will not necessarily meet with success, and consumers are then best protected by proper treatment of the wastes before application.

8
Planning and implementation

8.1 Resources planning

8.1.1 Wastes reuse and national development

The scarcity of surface and ground water in many countries has led, or is leading, to the development of national plans for the rational allocation, utilization and protection of all available water resources. The objective of such plans is to ensure, as far as is practically possible, the maximum economic yield from the use of a scarce resource. Human wastes are relevant to these national water plans as they can alter the physicochemical and microbiological quality of water and thus place restrictions on its use. The incorporation of wastes reuse planning protocols into national water plans is important, especially under conditions of water scarcity, not only to protect water quality but also to minimize treatment costs, to safeguard public health and to obtain the maximum possible agricultural and aquacultural benefit from the nutrients and organic matter contained in the wastes.

Once it is recognized that human wastes reuse is an integral part of national water resources development planning, it is possible to establish a national plan for wastes reuse. This will normally include plans to improve existing reuse practices as well as for new reuse programmes and projects. This section provides guidance on how such a plan may be established.

8.1.2 Institutional framework

At national level the use of wastewater and excreta is an activity that touches the responsibilities of several ministries or agencies. The principal ministerial responsibilities are usually more or less as follows, although some countries have different arrangements:

- **Ministry of Agriculture and Fisheries**: overall project planning; management of state-owned land; installation and operation of irrigation infrastructure; agricultural and aquacultural extension, including training; control of marketing.

- **Ministry of Health**: health protection, particularly establishment of quality standards, monitoring methods and schedules for treated excreta and wastewater; health education; disease surveillance and treatment.

- **Ministry of Water Resources**: integration of wastewater use into water resources planning and management.

- **Ministry of Public Works/Local Government**: excreta and wastewater collection and treatment.

- **Ministry of Finance and Economic Planning**: economic and financial appraisal of projects; import control (equipment, fertilizers).

Other ministries and government agencies, for example those concerned with environmental protection, land tenure, rural development, cooperatives and women's affairs, may also be involved. Unfortunately, the Ministry of Health is often only marginally involved in the sector, if at all, even where human wastes are used on a wide scale. Any effort to control the health risks from the practice will be greatly strengthened by the active participation of the Health Ministry. When implementing any new project or health protection measure that involves a change in farming practice, the Ministry of Agriculture will have a fundamental role to play.

Smooth cooperation between the relevant agencies is required, particularly between the technical staff involved. Some countries, especially those in which there are few natural water resources, may find it advantageous to establish an executive body, such as an interagency technical standing committee, under the aegis of a leading ministry (Agriculture or Water Resources), or possibly a separate parastatal organization (with both government and private capital) such as an Office for Wastewater Recycling (as in California, see Box 8.1), to be responsible for sector development, planning and management. Another approach (followed in Tunisia, see Box 8.2) is to include the promotion of waste recycling as a goal of the International Drinking Water Supply and Sanitation Decade, under an interministerial National Decade Coordinating Committee. Legal powers will be needed for this purpose.

Most countries, however, will not feel the need for such a formal arrangement, and a simple *ad hoc* committee will often suffice. Alternatively, existing organizations may be given responsibility for the sector, or parts of it; for example, a National Irrigation Board

---

Box 8.1 Wastewater use management in the United States of America

In the United States no single federal agency controls wastewater use, but several agencies have relevant responsibilities. The federal government has mandatory requirements on quality of sewage discharge, as well as providing grant funding for wastewater use projects. In this respect, the Environmental Protection Agency has the greatest influence on wastewater reclamations as its primary function is to enforce the provisions of the Federal Water Pollution Control Acts and other related federal legislation. Other federal agencies, such as the Bureau of Reclamation, have become involved in wastewater reclamation as a means of supplementing existing water resources.

On a state basis, the policies and agencies are varied, primarily as a result of varying views on the value of wastewater use as part of the overall resource. Perhaps the best example of a comprehensive state programme is that developed by California, where wastewater use is an integral part of water resource planning. In 1977 the State Water Resources Control Board adopted the Policy and Action Plan for Water Reclamation in California, which includes funding for projects that make beneficial use of wastewaters. The plan also includes guidelines for project implementation. In addition the Governor created an Office of Water Recycling within the State Board to promote wastewater use within the state. The Office has two committees: one is for interagency coordination, and the second is an advisory committee composed of representatives of the water community together with technical specialists. The state's Regional Water Quality Boards are responsible for coordination at the local level, including the evaluation of applications for wastewater use permits and the enforcement of any restrictions on wastewater use.

Source: Fordham (1984).

---

might be made responsible for wastewater use in agriculture, and a National Fisheries Board for the aquacultural use of excreta and wastewater. Such an organization should then convene a committee of representatives from the different agencies having sectoral responsibilities.

Setting up an interagency or interministerial committee involves a compromise between representatives at too high a level, who are often too busy to meet, and those at too junior a level, who are unable to take decisions or to ensure they are implemented. The most likely problem in the long term is that the committee will fail to meet regularly. Its terms of reference should therefore lay down a mini-

---

Box 8.2 Management of wastewater use in Tunisia

The Water Law, enacted in 1975, stipulates that water resource planning must start from the principle of making the fullest possible use of every cubic metre of water. This includes the use of all treated wastewater, which has been set by the National Sanitation Commission as one of the objectives for the Water Supply and Sanitation Decade.

Initial studies are carried out by ONAS (*Office Nationale de l'Assainissement*), the national sanitation agency, which has recently examined plans for 20 new schemes. Many of the schemes are on state-owned land (*terres domaniales*) occupied by tenant farmers. The construction of works to transport and distribute the treated wastewater from the treatment plant to the irrigated area is carried out by the Directorate of Hydraulic Works in the Ministry of Agriculture.

The system is then operated by local Agricultural Development Authorities, also under the Ministry of Agriculture, which charge for the water and have powers to fine or disconnect supplies to farmers who disobey crop restriction regulations.

Elsewhere, the Ministry of Agriculture may authorize private companies to manage wastewater irrigation schemes, as in one case where the management of a hotel complex is authorized to irrigate with the treated wastewater from the hotel. The authorization documents include a restriction to lawns (including a golf course), ornamental plants and non-fruit trees, as well as a set of provisions (a *cahier des charges*) specifying the rights and duties of the hotel management, the Ministry of Agriculture, ONAS and the Ministry of Public Health.

The Ministry of Public Health is responsible for the hygienic quality of the wastewater used for irrigation and of the crops marketed. It is also responsible for monitoring of water pollution and enforcement of pollution control regulations, and plays an important role in formulating the regulations affecting the use of wastewater.

Source: Strauss (1986b).

---

mum frequency for meetings, and this is most likely to be sustained if a single interested person or department is responsible for calling regular meetings and following up decisions.

In countries with a regional or federal administration, such arrangements for interagency collaboration will be still more important at regional or state level. Whereas the general framework of wastes use policy and standards may be defined at national level, the regional body will have to interpret and add to these in the light of local conditions. An example of this is the relationship between federal and state bodies in the United States (see Box 8.1).

With regard to health protection measures, the interministerial body's main tasks would be:

- to develop a coherent national or regional policy and monitor its implementation;

- to define the division of responsibilities between the respective ministries and other bodies involved in the sector, and the form of liaison between them;

- to appraise major proposed new schemes from the point of view of public health and environmental protection;

- to oversee the promotion and enforcement of national legislation and codes of practice;

- to develop a coherent manpower development policy for the sector.

The institutional framework at the level of the individual project is discussed in Section 8.3.4.

8.2 Improvement of existing practices

Human wastes are already used for crop and fish production in many countries, often illegally and without official recognition by the health authorities. Where the practice is traditional or has arisen spontaneously, untreated or insufficiently treated wastes are commonly used. Experience in many countries has shown that simply to ban the practice is not likely to have very much effect on its prevalence or on the public health risk involved. On the contrary, banning the practice does not necessarily stop it, but may make it more difficult to supervise and control, and may also interfere with disease surveillance and health care among those most exposed to the risk of infection. A more promising approach is to provide support to improve existing use practices, not only to minimize the health risks but also to increase productivity.

Some legal controls will usually be required as well. However, it is easier to make regulations than to enforce them. In drafting new regulations (or in choosing which existing ones to enforce) it is important to plan for the institutions, staff and resources necessary to ensure they are followed. Perhaps even more important is to ensure that the regulations are realistic and achievable in the context in which they are to be applied. It will often be advantageous to adopt a gradual approach, or to test a new set of regulations by persuading a local administration to pass them as by-laws before they are extended to the rest of the country.

Measures to protect public health are particularly difficult to implement when there are many individual sources or owners of the waste, whether these are individual septic tank overflows, nightsoil collectors, or farmers with riparian rights to pump from a river so polluted as to contain only slightly diluted sewage. If the waste can be brought under unified control by installing a sewerage system, by establishing a central nightsoil treatment plant or by diverting the sewage from the river to a treatment works, this will give the controlling body much greater power to influence the ways in which the waste is subsequently used, and thus to minimize the risk to health. As can be seen from these examples, the measures required to obtain this control will often amount in practice to setting up a new scheme. This is discussed in Section 8.3.

8.2.1 Surveys

The first stage in any effort to improve existing practices must be to find out what those practices are and on what scale they are to be found. Such practices are often illegal, or believed to be so, and therefore are not likely to be mentioned in official documentation. Moreover, farmers may not be willing to let officials know that they use wastewater or excreta, for fear of being prosecuted or possibly obliged to pay for the wastes they use. There is therefore no substitute for a diligent search for the practice in the field, combined with tactful informal conversations with farmers and local officials. Interested local bodies, such as farmers' associations, marketing organizations and nongovernmental community organizations, may sometimes be better informed than government officials.

A visit to all wastewater outlets and a short walk downstream from each of them will often reveal surprises, as will an inspection of nightsoil disposal sites. The staff at such sites and at sewage treatment works will usually be well aware of any agricultural or aquacultural use of wastes in the area. So also will health inspectors, though they may need to be reassured that, if they are unable to enforce regulations, this is not necessarily a reflection upon their competence, diligence or integrity.

Wastewater is often used informally after it has been discharged and diluted in a natural watercourse. The associated health risk may be practically the same as if undiluted wastewater had been used, especially when the natural flow in the river or stream is little more than the flow of sewage in the dry season (when the water is most likely to be used). In some cases, on-site excreta disposal systems are also involved. Overflowing effluent from septic tanks may be used to irrigate gardens and vegetable patches in urban areas, and latrine pits may be emptied informally to fertilize nearby fields or fishponds.

At this stage, the survey should be kept as informal and open-ended as possible. Later, when the principal questions are clear and quantitative data are needed, a structured interview of farmers may be used (see Simpson-Hebert, 1983).

The results of the survey may be surprising and possibly shocking, and a tempting response may be to enforce blanket prohibitions, especially where such regulations already exist. However, such action is likely to be ineffective and even counterproductive, and is best avoided until the policy alternatives described below have been carefully considered. It is also advisable to assess the health risks of any waste recycling practices in the context of general patterns of hygiene and disease transmission in the area. For example, faecal coliforms or *Ascaris* eggs may be found on vegetables fertilized by wastewater, but such contamination should be compared with that found on the same products, grown by other methods, at local points of sale such as markets. An epidemiological survey among farm workers may also help to put health risks in perspective (see Box 8.3). If the farm workers eat some of their own produce then they (and their families) are the group most exposed to the risk of infection.

An informal survey of reuse practices should aim not only to find out where wastes are being used, but also to answer the following questions:

- How are the wastes collected, treated and stored?

- What quantities are used?

- What quantities are available?

- On which crops are they applied?

- What are the benefits of using them?

- How and when are they applied?

Box 8.3 Assessment of health risks by epidemiological surveys

An epidemiological survey among farm workers would aim to assess the amount of disease caused by the practice of using human wastes. This can be done by comparing the level of disease in the 'exposed' population (which uses wastes) with that in an 'unexposed' or control population (which does not). The difference in disease levels may then be attributed to the practice of using the wastes, provided that the two populations compared are similar in all other respects including socioeconomic status and ethnic group.

It is best to restrict the study to the excreta-related diseases of most importance in farm workers locally. These will usually include intestinal helminth infections and diarrhoeal disease and, in some areas, typhoid fever and hepatitis A infection. Where aquaculture is practised, particular helminthic infections may be important, e.g. clonorchiasis, schistosomiasis.

The choice of infections for study and the method of study should also be guided by practical considerations. In a one-off, cross-sectional survey, the size of the sample needed will depend on the prevalence of the infection and on the difference in prevalence between the two groups that the study aims to detect. In general, large sample sizes are needed when the prevalence of the infection is low. This means that a study of the prevalence of diarrhoeal disease in farm workers will normally need a larger sample size than a study of intestinal helminth infections (for example, *Ascaris*, *Trichuris* and hookworm). The following two examples give an idea of the sample sizes required to have a 90% chance of detecting a difference at the 5% level of statistical significance:

- A sample size of about 230 per group would be needed where the prevalence of *Ascaris* infection in the general (unexposed) population is 30% and has been raised to 45% in the exposed population.

- About 1720 people would be needed in each group where the prevalence of diarrhoeal disease in the general (unexposed) population is 5% and has been raised to 7.5% in the exposed population.

Diarrhoeal disease is common but has a low prevalence at any given moment because of the short duration of each episode. For this case, the necessary sample size could be reduced by using a prospective cohort study, which monitors the incidence of disease over a period of time. This is, however, much more difficult to organize.

Sample sizes should be calculated with reference to appropriate

---

(Box 8.3 continued)

statistical texts (for example: Fleiss, 1981; Lwanga & Lemeshow, 1989) and by consulting WHO guidelines (for example, World Health Organization, 1981b).

An epidemiological survey is a complex undertaking and should involve trained staff in the Ministry of Health. The study should be led by an epidemiologist, and a statistician should be involved at an early stage to help in survey design as well as analysis of the data. A study will normally go through four phases:

1. the preparatory work, including study design and identification of the sample population and questionnaire development;

2. the pilot study, to judge the feasibility and appropriateness of the study, train field workers and refine the questionnaire;

3. the field work proper;

4. analysis of the data.

Guidelines on the conduct and interpretation of studies in environmental epidemiology have been published by WHO (1983). Although these guidelines deal mainly with the effect of chemicals and with chronic disease, they are also very relevant to studies of the effect of wastes reuse on infectious diseases.

Source: U. Blumenthal, personal communication.

Answers to the last question may suggest possible interventions. Some aspects of the existing practice may already help to reduce the health risk — for instance when nightsoil is buried before planting — and these can provide a basis for further improvements.

It will also be helpful to examine the organizational setting. The farmers may own the land, or they may be employees, tenants, share-croppers or squatters. They may or may not be free in practice to choose their crop or their agricultural (or aquacultural) methods, because of their status or because of marketing constraints. If health risks are to be reduced, someone will have to be persuaded, induced or obliged to change the present practice, and this may not necessarily be the person working in the field.

8.2.2 Existing regulations

If it is considered that the use of human wastes in agriculture or aquaculture is posing a health risk, it will be useful to study the existing relevant legislation and regulations before considering the policy options to minimize that risk. These will include the Water Law, where it exists, as well as legislation on environmental pollution, water quality, food hygiene and occupational health.

In many cases it will be found that this legislation is regularly being flouted, especially where there are strong economic motives for doing so. This can happen, for example, near large cities in arid regions, where the city wastewater may be a priceless resource not so much because it contains wastes but rather because it is almost the only water available. Farmers in such areas have been known to break open sewers to divert raw wastewater on to their land. In areas of high population density the production of crops, and sometimes fish, is often so intense that every hectare must produce the maximum amount possible. Excreta then become very valuable because of their nutrient content. In parts of Asia, for example, it has been known for the contents of a latrine to be stolen at night for use in agriculture.

When human wastes become valuable, whether because of the water that carries them or for the nutrients they contain, farmers will wish to use such a precious resource on the most profitable crop. Where the farmers are poor or lack secure tenure of the land, an additional factor in their choice of crop may be their need for a quick return on the money they invest. A squatter, for example, cannot usually wait for fruit trees to mature, lest he be evicted and the site bulldozed for a new building. The crop will therefore often be a vegetable crop and it may sometimes be eaten raw.

Where current reuse practice contravenes existing regulations, it is important to investigate the reasons why these regulations are not being enforced. Unless the various reasons for non-enforcement, outlined below, can be eliminated, future legislation is likely to fare no better.

Inappropriate standards

Rightly or wrongly there may be a general consensus that there is no serious health risk or that to enforce the regulations will not significantly reduce it. Alternatively, there may be ignorance of measures to minimize the health risk other than those that would seriously prejudice the farmers' income. If there is in fact no health risk, there is no need for enforcement. If there is a risk, then motivation of enforcement staff by educating them about the existing health risk and training them in low-cost ways to minimize it should become a priority.

In many cases, regulations such as wastewater quality standards have been borrowed from other countries with no consideration of their suitability for local conditions. Others have been adopted for reasons quite unconnected with epidemiological evidence of whether or not they are necessary. For example the only state in the USA that has adopted a virological standard of wastewater quality for reuse happens to have a university that has developed techniques for the virological examination of wastewater.

The thoughtless borrowing or introduction of over-stringent regulations can have one of two outcomes. Either the regulations will be flouted, creating the same health risks as if they did not exist; or they will cause an unnecessary fear of prosecution or disease and thus squander resources by discouraging all use of human wastes. A more realistic set of standards, which are totally adequate to safeguard public health, would be based on the Engelberg guideline values (see Tables 1.4 and 1.6).

Ignorance of the relevant legislation

This is best dealt with by education and training of the enforcement staff.

Lack of resources

It is usually a job for health inspectors to ensure that, where it is permitted, the use of wastes to produce crops or fish is carried out in a hygienic manner as prescribed by law. In some cases, the Ministry of Agriculture or the authority that manages a wastewater irrigation system may be responsible for applying crop restrictions or for otherwise regulating agricultural practices. Whichever arrangement has been adopted, the relevant body must rely on its field staff to police the regulations that it administers. Field staff, however, are likely to have so many other pressing tasks that this one is neglected, or they may lack the means of transport required to make regular visits to the area.

It is arguably a good idea for the role of enforcement officer to be combined with that of extension agent or irrigation system manager. This will ensure that staff are in the area regularly, and also help the farmers to see them as colleagues rather than as opponents. However, more staff may be needed if health risks are to be controlled.

Lack of definition of responsibilities

Often, however, the problem is not so much a shortage of field staff as a lack of definition of who is to enforce the rules, of the degree of priority this task should have in job descriptions, and of how staff are to be supervised and called to account in the performance of this duty.

External pressure

A common problem is the tendency of prominent local citizens, who may own large areas of land or fish ponds, to try to use their influence to avoid the sanctions of the law. After a few such cases, enforcement officers such as health inspectors may give up trying, because it may be risky for them to prosecute such people. The problem is most likely to occur where the cost of compliance with the regulations is relatively high. The rate of compliance may be increased by relaxing the regulations, or by actively enforcing only those regulations that can be met relatively easily. An alternative approach, where the rules cannot be relaxed without an unacceptable health risk, is to bring the enforcement officers under close supervision from a higher level. A senior official from a national body is less likely to be suborned or intimidated than a health assistant employed by a local municipality.

8.2.3 Policy options

The available technical measures that can be taken to avoid the health risks of using wastes have been outlined in Section 7. In practice, in a context where excreta or wastewater is already being used, not all of these measures will be feasible or appropriate, and the choice of the most appropriate combination will depend on local circumstances.

It is advisable to start by choosing a few practical and possibly quite modest steps, which can be taken with the available resources, to give a progressive improvement in the situation. They could be implemented one by one, or tried in one area before being extended progressively until overall coverage is achieved. Whatever the coverage or time-scale involved, their implementation should be monitored to ensure that they are achievable and to rectify any mistakes.

The following sections consider the managerial factors relevant to the feasibility, planning and implementation of the available options. For each type of use, these are discussed under the headings used in Section 7, that is: treatment, crop restriction, application, and human exposure control.

Treatment

Wastewater. Treatment is an option that involves few technical problems when the wastewater collected by a sewerage system is to be used for irrigation. Its drawback is that it usually requires a substantial capital investment, although upgrading or improving the operation of existing wastewater treatment plants can sometimes be cheap and effective (see Section 7.2.5).

The building of a wastewater treatment plant on the most suitable available land will often alter the place where the wastewater is discharged. This will benefit the owners or occupiers of land near the new discharge site, while others may lose. It will be necessary to make some concessions to the latter if their cooperation is required; aggrieved farmers have been known to break open the sewers upstream of a new treatment plant so as not to lose their access to the raw sewage.

The land where untreated wastewater is used for agriculture will often be the most suitable land for the treatment plant, but its location on the outskirts of a city also makes it very desirable for building as the city expands. Indeed, it may already have been bought by speculators. If it is still in the hands of those who farm it, a strong inducement for them to sell at a reasonable price may be an offer of downstream land and water rights to allow them to continue using the treated effluent from the new plant.

Much uncontrolled use of wastewater is by abstraction from rivers that are so heavily polluted as to consist of only slightly diluted raw sewage. Sometimes it may be more feasible to cover the river as a sewer and treat the full flow, rather than to collect or treat the many small discharges into it. If it is decided to introduce or improve the treatment of wastewater discharged into such a river, consideration should be given to setting up a formal irrigation scheme to use the wastewater. This gives control of the wastewater and its use to a single authority, which greatly simplifies the implementation of other measures for health protection, as will be seen in the following paragraphs. The planning and implementation of such a scheme are further discussed in Section 8.3.

Treatment is a much harder option to implement when the wastewater in use comes from a variety of sources, such as over-flowing septic tanks. One approach may be to take action against those who produce the wastewater, to prevent the environmental pollution it causes. The owners of septic tanks, for example, could be obliged to build adequate soakaways and desludge the tanks to prevent blockage of those soakaways that still function. Even then, the safe use of the wastewater is not necessarily ruled out. The subsoil irrigation provided by soakaways may sustain hygienic and profitable small-scale urban agriculture in the gardens where they are located.

In other cases, the only solution may be to build major sanitation works. When large numbers of septic tanks overflow, for example, it may indicate that there is not enough room, in the circumstances, to build adequate soakaways: a small-bore sewerage network (Otis & Mara, 1985) is needed to collect the effluent. The effluent can then be treated in a single treatment works, thus greatly simplifying the technical and organizational aspects of treatment and subsequent reuse.

Excreta. In the same way, treatment of excreta is much more readily implemented where a single body such as a municipality collects the excreta and can also manage the treatment process. Careful supervision may be needed so that treatment — often a prolonged process — is carried out for the full period required. Otherwise, at times of great demand, it can be tempting to take short-cuts and allow the use of partially treated excreta.

When excreta from many small sources is used, it is rather harder to institute treatment separately at all of these sources. In some large Asian cities, where nightsoil is collected by many small entrepreneurs for sale to farmers on the outskirts, it might be possible for a municipal body to purchase the raw nightsoil from them and sell the treated product back to them. Since composted nightsoil is a more effective fertilizer, it may be possible to sell it for a slightly higher price, the difference going towards the cost of composting.

In rural areas, however, farmers who have used raw excreta for years will not be easily persuaded to treat it. They may find it hard to believe that such a long-established practice is harmful to their health. A more persuasive approach may be to show them, by the use of local demonstration plots, that higher crop yields are obtained with treated excreta. This is a job for the agricultural extension service.

Of course, for the agricultural extension officers to have a chance of success, the treated excreta must in fact be more effective and not too unattractive to use. Farmers may be discouraged from using excreta composted with solid waste if it contains large undigested items of debris from the solid waste. It may therefore be necessary to remove such debris from the compost to make it saleable.

Aquaculture. In traditional aquaculture using wastewater or excreta, treatment is probably the option most likely to succeed. One treatment option for aquaculture is to connect ponds in series (or to divide a pond into compartments connected in series) and avoid harvesting from the first pond. Existing ponds connected in series may have different owners, so that to promote this option it may be necessary to establish cooperative arrangements between them. Another approach may be to establish an uncontaminated depuration pond in which the fish are kept for several weeks before harvesting. This can be done by building a new pond, or by separating off part of an existing one.

Whatever method is used for health protection when using excreta in aquaculture, its implementation is likely to demand a change in behaviour, and probably the expenditure of money, by a large number of individual users, and again an additional motive is probably required. One such motivating factor might be the greater convenience and privacy of an inhouse toilet, the waste from which can be treated, compared with an overhung latrine over a fish pond.

Crop restriction

Crop restriction is relatively simple to implement where the wastes are used by a small number of large bodies, whether they are private firms, cooperatives, state farms, or the municipal authority itself. However, the enforcement of crop restrictions on a large number of small farmers is much more difficult. The edible crops most likely to be excluded, such as salad vegetables, are among those with the highest cash yields. There may be a good market for them in the nearby urban community producing the wastewater, and moreover their short growing season gives a relatively quick return on the cash invested by comparison with, say, fruit trees.

Crop restrictions are not impossible in such circumstances; they are most likely to succeed where local dietary habits limit the demand for uncooked vegetables, and where there are profitable alternative crops such as cereals, for which a market exists (see Box 8.4). Industrial crops, such as cotton, or grapes for wine production, can be particularly suitable for cultivation under crop restrictions (see Box 8.5).

In some countries, the existing agricultural planning machinery allows a firm control of all crops grown, with regular inspection of every farmer's fields and sanctions against those who depart from the plan. These arrangements can be used at little extra cost to ensure that crop restrictions are followed.

If there is no local experience of the application of crop restrictions, their feasibility should be tested in a trial area before they are

Box 8.4 Crop restriction in Irrigation District 03, Mexico

Where irrigation water contains untreated sewage, as occurs in District 03, national regulations restrict the crops grown to those that are eaten cooked, those eaten uncooked but which do not come into contact with the soil, and fodder crops. In each irrigation district, a local committee consisting of representatives of the Department of Agriculture and Water Resources (SARH) and of local groups makes agreements on water distribution, crop restrictions and cropping patterns. In District 03, the committee includes representatives from the local agriculture secretariat, local banks, agricultural industries, marketing groups, farm owners and cooperative farm workers, as well as members from SARH.

Prohibited crops include lettuce, cabbage, carrots, radishes, beet, coriander, spinach and parsley. The main crops grown are shown in the table below.

Crop	Area cultivated (ha)	Percentage of total	Water requirement (cm)	Net profit per hectare ($\times$ 1000 pesos)
Maize	19 668	41.0	100	41.4
Alfalfa	17 972	37.5	158	22.4
Barley	1 852	3.9	72	15.8
Oats	1 706	3.6	72	4.0
Wheat	458	1.0	113	11.6
Chillies	999	2.1	108	154.9
Green tomatoes	587	1.2	141	192.5
Haricot beans	865	1.8	31	20.1
Broad beans	301	0.6	88	18.3
Others	3 574	7.3	97	58.6

The first five crops in the table are cereals and fodder crops, and account for 87% of the total area under cultivation. Compliance with the crop restrictions is enforced by SARH personnel in charge of each section of the District. However, because of the great demand for maize (the staple food) and fodder crops in Mexico, and since raw vegetables do not form a major part of the diet of most people, non-compliance with the restrictions is not a serious problem. Farmers are allowed to grow chillies and green tomatoes, which although they are eaten raw grow well above the ground and are therefore not usually contaminated by sewage used in surface irrigation. There is a strong demand by the farmers to grow these crops, because of their importance in the Mexican diet and their high economic return.

Source: U. Blumenthal, personal communication.

Box 8.5 Crop restriction in Ica, Peru

The town of Ica lies on the coast of Peru about 300 km south of Lima, and is surrounded by desert. It was traditionally a wine-producing area, but cotton began to compete with grapes in the early 1900s. Irrigation water was initially obtained from rivers and wells, but now wastewater is also used.

The majority of the sewage from Ica is treated in four waste stabilization ponds at Cachiche. However, the ponds are unfortunately connected in parallel and therefore produce a relatively poor quality effluent, with a faecal coliform concentration of about $10^5/100$ ml. This effluent is used to irrigate about 400 hectares of land; because of the poor quality of the effluent, the cultivation of tubers and other vegetables that grow close to the ground, or that are consumed raw, is not permitted. The major crops grown are cotton, maize, and grapes. In addition, the sewage from Tinguina, a suburb of Ica, is treated in a single waste stabilization pond. The effluent is used to irrigate a further 130 hectares, where mainly cotton and fruit trees are grown. Near to these areas, ground water is used to irrigate vegetables and other crops that cannot be grown using the wastewater.

The successful operation of the ponds, use of the effluent and enforcement of crop restrictions can be explained by several factors: the history of cultivation of non-vegetable crops in the area, the availability of ground water to enable some farmers in the area to grow vegetables, and cooperation between the Water and Sewerage Service, which operates the sewage treatment ponds, and the Health Inspectorate, which enforces the regulations.

Source: U. Blumenthal, personal communication.

implemented on a wide scale. The trial will also give an initial estimate of the resources required for enforcement, as well as clarifying the most suitable institutional arrangements for implementation of restrictions. These should include arrangements for marketing those crops that are permitted, at a high enough price to interest the farmers. Where greater cash inputs or a longer growing season are involved, assisted access to agricultural credit may also be necessary.

Enforcement at the field may not always be as easy as might at first appear. Though a crop may take months to grow and can be inspected throughout this time, the wastewater may need to be applied for only a few days each month, and this can be concealed even from vigilant inspectors. Some of the lessons learned from the successful crop restriction system in Mexico are summarized in Box 8.6.

Another approach might be to monitor the microbiological quality of food sold at the market, although this has never been used in practice to enforce crop restrictions and would face several difficulties. First, a considerable amount of experimentation would be required to define achievable standards of quality. An *a priori* standard may not be met even by produce grown without the use of wastes, and any attempt to enforce it would be self-defeating. Second, it is not always easy to trace the origins of a consignment of agricultural produce sampled on a market stall, and less so when the results of microbiological examination are known, a day or two after sampling. Third, regular sampling from the many places where foodstuffs are sold would require laboratories with the capacity to analyse a formidable number of samples. On the other hand the collection of a few samples from market stalls for examination, with a possible threat of action against those producing or selling heavily contaminated foodstuffs, could have a salutary effect on food hygiene generally, including crops grown using wastes in areas unknown to the health authorities.

Box 8.6 Enforcement of crop restrictions

Crop restrictions have been enforced over many decades in the areas irrigated with wastewater from Mexico City. This experience has shown the need for a comprehensive programme to ensure compliance with the regulations, which should include the following principal components.

(a) A small but flexible and efficient inspection and regulatory service with well trained personnel able to identify the banned crops and the location of risk areas in terms of wastewater quality. Staff of this regulatory service must be instructed to perform their duties with dignity and honesty, trying to be advisors and educators rather than policemen. The use of an inspection operating manual and standardized forms is desirable. Under normal conditions, the immediate responsibility for successful implementation of crop regulations rests upon those in charge of irrigation permits and also upon the extension agents.

(b) The issue of permits based on a complete inventory of land and farms using wastewater. The permit form should include such data as name, land location, surface to be irrigated, water re-

(Box 8.6 continued)

quired and manner of application, crops and marketing arrangements. Permits should be renewable after each crop cycle.

(c) A well organized training programme with provisions for selecting manpower. Emphasis must be placed on the employment of professional personnel including sanitary engineers.

(d) Information on the crop regulations must be effectively disseminated. Wide publicity is required to alert enforcement staff, farmers and the public in general of the health risk involved in raw wastewater, the reasons why crops have to be controlled, and the need for their participation. The general public must be educated to recognize the need for these public health regulations, with greater public concern for improved public health and safer food production.

(e) The integration of activities necessitates cooperation and coordination among government agencies such as public health, agriculture, livestock and water authorities, at national, state and local levels. Trade and transportation authorities must be informed of the crop regulations related to places of crop production from sewage farms and the prohibited categories.

(f) To be effective, the regulatory agency and its activities must be established by law and firmly supported by law enforcement organizations. A legal advisory service is needed.

(g) Provision must be made for detecting and monitoring the microbiological and chemical quality of water, soil and crops. This requires adequate laboratory facilities for analytical work.

(h) The irrigation district should maintain up-to-date farm control records with periodic evaluation of data on excreta-related diseases.

(i) The entire crop control system requires careful technical and administrative supervision to ensure, for instance, that no inspectors succumb to corruption, as this would render it useless.

(j) Office support facilities and transportation are indispensable for the implementation of the programme.

Source: Romero (1987).

Application

Wastewater. Irrigation by sprinkler demands careful measures for the protection of the workforce and nearby residents from exposure to infection. However, sprinkler irrigation is unlikely to be practised except in large, centralized schemes run by a single body which is in a relatively good position to ensure that these other measures are implemented.

A change in an existing wastewater irrigation method to reduce health risks is most likely to be needed when the current practice is flooding. Farmers may not be very enthusiastic about the alternative (for instance furrow irrigation), as it is likely to involve them in additional work and expense. They may need help with levelling of the land and possibly with contour ploughing to create the furrows. The change will also help to reduce mosquito breeding and other forms of exposure to disease occasioned by wading in areas flooded with wastewater. In addition to the diminished risk to farmers' health, arguments that may persuade them to change might include the greater efficiency of other irrigation methods when limited quantities of water are available, and the reduced mosquito nuisance. The Agricultural Extension Service is best placed to encourage farmers to change their irrigation methods. Its task will be easier if a high enough charge is levied for the wastewater to encourage its efficient use.

Subsurface or localized (drip, trickle or bubbler) irrigation can give a still greater degree of protection from contamination as well as using water more efficiently and often producing higher yields. It is expensive, however, and has not yet been used on a wide scale for irrigation with wastewater. A high degree of reliable treatment is required, to prevent clogging of the small holes (emitters) through which water is slowly released into the soil, although this is not a problem with bubbler irrigation.

Excreta. As is the case for wastewater, the Agricultural Extension Service may be in the best position to promote hygienic practices relating to the application of excreta. Where a municipal body controls the source of nightsoil, it may be able to encourage application before the start of the growing season by making the nightsoil available only at certain times of the year. Alternatively, the agency controlling distribution of the nightsoil may itself apply it to the farmers' fields and charge them for this service. The workers handling the excreta will then be the employees of a single body, which will facilitate exposure control measures among them.

Human exposure control

Measures to reduce exposure to diarrhoeal diseases generally and to promote good case management are well known components of primary health care. They include health education, particularly regarding domestic hygiene and breast-feeding, and the promotion of oral rehydration solutions prepared from sachets or from ingredients available in the home.

An obvious measure is to provide an adequate water supply and sanitation. Controlling the exposure of agricultural workers to faecal contamination in the fields may have little effect if they continue to be exposed to infection from their drinking-water and in their home environment through lack of these basic facilities. Particular care is required to ensure that the use of human wastes does not cause contamination of nearby wells or other sources of drinking-water

Where salaried agricultural workers are involved, their employers have a responsibility to protect them from exposure to diseases, which in many countries is set down in existing legislation on occupational health. This may need to be brought to the employers' attention, together with guidance on the measures they should take such as the issuing of protective clothing, particularly footwear. Employers often despair of issuing footwear, claiming that their workers do not use it, or that they sell it or save it to wear on special occasions. Any effort to promote the issuing of protective clothing by employers must be accompanied by still greater efforts to convince their employees that they must wear it.

Measures to control the exposure of those who handle the crops can be implemented in much the same way as for farm-workers. When they all work for a small number of employers, exposure control fits into a general programme of occupational health. On the other hand, when a large number of petty traders are involved, selling or making products from the crops, it will be difficult to implement exposure control measures unless they are all gathered together in a market. Most markets are in any case subject to public health inspection, and basic exposure control measures may be a good thing whether or not crops produced using wastes are being handled. As well as protecting crop-handlers from contamination, they may also help to protect other crops from contamination by the handlers.

Markets may also be the best places to advise consumers about the hygienic precautions they should take with the produce they purchase. It is certainly good for consumers to be told of anything they can do to protect themselves from exposure to infection. However, they cannot be relied upon to do it, especially where it would mean a change from long-standing habits.

Residents who are not involved in the use of wastewater or excreta are best placed to ensure that their health is not put at risk by those who are, once it has been explained to them what precautions are required and what risks they and their families may run if the precautions are not taken. Of course, a government inspector can ensure that fences are built and warning signs put up, but vigilant neighbours will be the first to notice when they need repair or replacement or when sprinkler irrigation begins to encroach on land too close to their homes. The establishment of a residents' health committee can be a focus for a health education campaign, as well as providing a locally controlled institution to monitor the practice of wastes reuse.

Treatment (chemotherapy) of agricultural workers, their families and other exposed groups for intestinal helminth infections is relatively easy to administer in a formal wastewater irrigation scheme, although additional health personnel may be required to treat a large population. It can be quite popular, and provides an excellent opportunity for follow-up with hygiene education activities to publicize simple measures for personal protection. The cost of chemotherapy may be paid by the employers where salaried workers or share-croppers work the fields, or paid for out of the fees charged for irrigation permits where these are used.

Where wastewater is used on many small and scattered farms, there are greater logistic problems and the identification and treatment of exposed persons may become quite expensive. An additional problem arises where the wastewater is used illegally, as farmers may be unwilling to come forward, fearing prosecution. It may be necessary to give them reassurance by proclaiming an amnesty and by using different health personnel for the chemotherapy programme from those responsible for enforcing the sanitary regulations.

Those living close to irrigated fields or ponds are likely to include farm workers and their families, who will be exposed to infection in several ways. It may be easier to include them all in a mass treatment campaign aimed at farm workers than to attempt to determine the employment status of each individual.

The identification of infected individuals for treatment can be costly and time-consuming. Where the prevalence of infection is relatively high, mass treatment of the whole exposed population may be worth while. Against this must be set the cost of unnecessary treatment of persons who are not infected. The choice between mass chemotherapy and selective chemotherapy of infected individuals therefore depends largely on the prevalence of infection and on the relative costs of detection and treatment of cases.

Costs

The choice of which of these options to implement must be based not only on their efficacy, but also on their cost. If the cost of those chosen for implementation is likely to exceed the economic benefit of using the wastes, it is important to consider whether less expensive measures might suffice, or whether it is worth while to use the wastes at all. In most cases, the benefits are likely to justify the costs, but some financial arrangement is needed to ensure that the costs are met from a suitable source. These aspects are considered in Section 8.4.

8.3 New schemes

8.3.1 Project identification

Upgrading of existing schemes should generally take priority over the development of new ones. Upgrading may be needed to improve agricultural or aquacultural yields or to reduce health risks. Attention should be paid not only to the technical improvements required (see Section 7.2.5), but also to the need for better management of schemes and to their improved operation and maintenance.

Ideally, new schemes should be identified and their relative priority established in the context of a national plan for wastewater and excreta use. However, opportunities for new schemes will often arise in connection with major wastewater construction projects, and these need not necessarily be rejected for lack of a national plan that includes them. On the contrary, the possibility of wastes reuse is always worth considering when drawing up plans for land use, housing development or waste management, and an assessment of prospects for waste reuse should be included in consultants' terms of reference.

On the other hand, new schemes should be viable, with a potentially good rate of agricultural or aquacultural return at minimal risk to health and at least cost. There should also be at least the potential for developing a satisfactory local institutional framework within which they can be properly planned, implemented and operated.

Outline planning should be done at the project identification stage. This involves determining the size and scope of the project, and needs data and preliminary decisions on the following aspects:

- available quantities and qualities of excreta/wastewater;

- land/pond area requirements;

- crops/fish to be grown;

- quality requirements for excreta/wastewater, and hence possible need for treatment;

- outline design for transportation of excreta/wastewater; storage requirements;

- preliminary selection of application techniques;

- institutional and organizational aspects;

- current legislation and regulations affecting the use of wastes;

- preliminary economic and financial justification for the projects, including details of the market for the product;

- project timetable;

- whether a pilot project is required.

The strategy to be adopted for health protection (see Section 7) should be an integral part of these considerations. Many of the policy aspects that apply to the improvement of an existing practice (see Section 8.2) should also be borne in mind when contemplating a new scheme. A preliminary environmental examination, and outline consideration of the principal environmental consequences of the project, are also advisable at this stage.

8.3.2 Pilot projects

A pilot project is particularly necessary in countries with little or no experience of the planned use of excreta or wastewater, or when the introduction of new techniques (for example, localized irrigation) is envisaged. The problem of health protection is only one of a number of interconnected questions that are difficult to answer without local experience of the kind a pilot project can give. These questions are likely to include important technical and economic aspects, including the feasibility of the scheme itself, so that preliminary trials on a pilot scale will often be essential anyway. A pilot scheme can also help to identify any potential health risks and develop ways to control them.

Proposals to introduce agricultural or aquacultural use of wastes are often made in connection with new sanitation works, particularly new wastewater treatment plants, but a pilot project at a nearby existing plant may provide the necessary advance information.

In parts of the world where a new scheme is most likely to be economically viable, it is especially probable that human wastes are already being used in some way or other. It will be well worth while to study existing practice in the area, and possibly in neighbouring countries, before considering new projects. Indeed, a government should at least consider how to ensure that the current practices are not hazardous to health before embarking on new developments in the sector.

From the agricultural (or aquacultural) point of view, a pilot project serves not only for experiment but also for demonstration. A representative selection of local or exotic crops should be made, and the experimental design should be a randomized complete block with at least three replications.

In the case of irrigation with treated wastewater or settled nightsoil, freshwater controls both with and without supplementary inorganic fertilizers are required; the use of diluted wastewater or nightsoil may be required for nitrogen-sensitive crops if nitrogen concentrations are high. Composted or thermophilically digested excreta, if used, should be applied to the experimental plots before planting, as should trenched nightsoil. Aquacultural pilot projects should be similarly planned: new fish species or plant crops should be investigated, with different application rates of different wastes (for example, pond effluents, compost, latrine contents). Information is required not only on crop yields but also on microbiological contamination levels, uptake of heavy metals, and soil and groundwater effects.

A pilot project should operate for at least one growing season, or at least one year if both winter and summer crops are to be investigated. It must be very carefully planned so that the work involved is not underestimated and can be carried out correctly; otherwise, repetition in the following year is required. After the experimental period, a successful pilot project may be translated into a demonstration project with training facilities for local operators and farmers.

8.3.3 Project planning: technical aspects

Detailed planning for excreta and wastewater use schemes should follow the usual national procedures for agricultural and aquacultural project planning, supplemented as necessary by the requirements of external funding agencies. The following discussion is centred on the particular planning needs resulting from the fact that the project is for excreta and/or wastewater use and from the need for health protection measures. In other regards, planning requirements for excreta and wastewater use schemes are similar to those for irrigation and fertilization schemes that are not based on the use of human wastes.

A great deal of information needs to be collected, and many decisions must be taken to prepare a detailed plan for a new scheme. The main technical aspects that should be covered by the plan are listed in Box 8.7. Several of these aspects interact. For example: in an irrigation scheme the types of crops affect the seasonal pattern of irrigation and hence the storage requirements; forestry can benefit from irrigation with wastewater at times when it is not required for other crops, and so help to balance the demand.

For each scheme, the planner should seek to maximize the net annual benefit from crop production in a manner consistent with labour constraints and the need to protect health and minimize costs. For this purpose it will be necessary to make cost estimates for the various activities, including major construction works for storage, treatment or transport of wastes, land preparation and irrigation infrastructure, and also for staffing, treatment, pumping and maintenance as well as other agricultural inputs.

An assessment of the benefits requires a forecast not only of the probable yields of the crops to be grown but also of their anticipated prices. This in turn demands a survey to establish that an adequate market exists for these crops. This is particularly important where crop restriction is to be employed as a health protection measure, and where the crops to be grown require industrial processing; in the latter case, sufficient processing capacity must be available.

Projects for the reuse of wastes are not static; they take time to be implemented and thereafter to evolve and grow. The plan should allow reasonable time-scales for all its aspects: to obtain funding, to execute any necessary construction works and to prepare the ground for the scheme to begin. From then onwards it should envisage the configuration of the project in each year of its future existence. For irrigation projects, a 20-year planning horizon is often considered.

Box 8.7 Technical information to be included in a project plan

Wastewater irrigation

- Current and predicted wastewater generation rates; current and predicted proportions of industrial effluents; degree of dilution by surface water.

- Existing and required wastewater treatment facilities; pathogen removal efficiencies, physicochemical quality.

- Irrigable land area: extent, location, type (virgin land, existing farmland, public parks); soil types, drainage, ground slopes (maps are needed).

- Local geology and potential risk of groundwater pollution.

- Conveyance of wastewater to the fields; pumping stations.

- Wastewater storage requirements, based on possible need to restrict irrigation to daytime or night-time, to utilize excess wastewater from a season that does not require it (for example, the rainy season), or to keep wastewater from one season to another to permit the production of more valuable or export crops, or crops that require greater wastewater treatment; or arrangements for wastewater disposal (if only dry-season irrigation is envisaged).

- Wastewater application methods for both restricted and unrestricted irrigation.

- Disposal of drainage waters, or their use to irrigate salt-resistant crops.

- Mix of crops to be irrigated; treatment implications of their wastewater quality requirements; if different qualities are required, how this can be achieved (for example, facultative pond effluent might be used for restricted irrigation, and maturation pond effluent for unrestricted irrigation).

- Crop water and supplementary nutrient requirements; crop nitrogen and boron sensitivities; soil leaching requirements.

- Estimated crop yields per hectare.

- Overall strategy for health protection.

(Box 8.7 continued)

Agricultural fertilization with excreta

- Current and predicted excreta/sludge generation rates.

- Existing and required treatment facilities; pathogen removal efficiencies, physicochemical quality.

- Fertilizable land area: extent, location, soil types.

- Conveyance of treated or raw excreta/sludge to the fields (collection by farmers or delivery by treatment authority).

- Excreta/sludge storage requirements.

- Excreta/sludge application rates and methods.

- Mix of crops to be fertilized, and their requirements for excreta/sludge quality, supplementary nutrients and water; treatment implications.

- Estimated crop yields per hectare.

- Strategy for health protection.

Aquacultural use of excreta and wastewater

- Current and projected generation rates of the wastes (excreta, sludge or wastewater); proportion of industrial effluents; dilution by surface water.

- Existing and required waste treatment facilities; pathogen removal efficiencies, physicochemical quality.

- Existing and required pond areas: size, location, soil types (lining requirements); depuration pond requirements.

- Evaporation (need for make-up water).

- Conveyance of treated wastes to ponds (collection of treated excreta and sludge by farmers or delivery by treatment authority).

- Storage requirements for the wastes.

- Waste application rates and methods.

(Box 8.7 continued)

- Types of fish and aquatic plants to be cultured, and their require-ments for wastes quality and supplementary nutrients.

- Estimated yields of fish or plants per hectare of pond per year.

- Feasibility of rearing ducks on the ponds; feeding requirements.

- Strategy for health protection.

It will often be advisable to allow for a modest beginning, followed by a phased expansion of the project in subsequent years (see Box 8.8). This will allow time to train farmers and staff in new methods and for lessons learnt in the early stages to influence later devel-opments. It will also help to ensure that the level of production does not over-reach the current availability of the waste or the demand for the crops produced.

Projects using wastewater will be affected by a progressive change not only in the quantity of wastewater available but also in its quality. As the number of people served by the sewerage network increases, this will lead to increased wastewater flows, to reduced dilution by storm water and by ground water infiltrating into sewers, and also to reduced retention times in wastewater treatment works. Where a new sewerage network has been built, the proportion of the popu-lation having connections to it may initially be very low indeed, and allowance for this should be made in the project plan.

Multiple use of wastes

The feasibility of integrated schemes making multiple use of wastes should also be considered, as this will often lead to reduced costs. For example: when wastewater from a series of stabilization ponds is used for irrigation, fish may be reared in the third and subsequent ponds in the series; excreta and sludge treatment facilities can often be located at a wastewater treatment works, and the treated product applied to the same fields that are irrigated with treated wastewater (although care must be taken not to overload the system with nutrients, especially nitrogen); aquaculture pond effluents may be used for crop irrigation. Biogas generation can also be linked to other uses for wastes, if there is a local demand for the gas.

> ## Box 8.8 Wastewater irrigation in Kuwait
>
> Wastewater irrigation in Kuwait started on a limited scale in the mid-1970s, with alfalfa grown as the main crop to feed cattle for the dairy industry. On the basis of the experience gained, the first phase of expansion was commissioned ten years later, bringing the total farm area to over 1700 ha. Garlic and onions will also be grown, like the alfalfa, under sprinkler irrigation. Aubergines and peppers will be irrigated using flood and furrow techniques.
>
> The scheme will be further extended as the available quantity of treated wastewater increases. It aims to make Kuwait self-sufficient in milk, potatoes, onions and garlic by the year 2010. In addition, an ambitious afforestation programme is planned, to provide wind and dust breaks along major highways and to protect new townships.
>
> All areas where wastewater is applied are fenced off to prevent public access, and farm workers are to be subjected to regular health checks. One factor permitting the efficient organization of the health protection strategy and of the project as a whole is that the farm is managed by a single company, which is supplied with treated wastewater by the Ministry of Public Works.
>
> *Source:* Cowan & Johnson (1985).

8.3.4 Project planning: institutional aspects

A detailed discussion on the organization of irrigation schemes is given in a recent FAO publication (Sagardoy, 1982), and much of it is applicable to the organization of schemes for the agricultural use of excreta and the aquacultural use of excreta and wastewater. The following discussion focuses on those aspects particularly relevant to such schemes.

To a substantial degree the organizational pattern of a wastes reuse scheme will be determined by the established land use pattern and existing institutions. Health protection measures are easier to implement effectively when the scheme is run as a single unit, whether by a private company, by a cooperative or by a public body (see Box 8.8). However, where the land involved is already farmed by smallholders, it will usually be unavoidable that they should continue to farm it when the use of wastes is introduced. In this case, some form of users' association and a joint management board would be almost essential for the implementation of those health protection measures that require their cooperation.

It may also be necessary to give the smallholders some security of tenure of the land and of their right to the wastewater in appropriate quantities and at appropriate times, especially if they are to be required to invest more cash or to change to crops that take longer to mature. This may be difficult when the owners of the land have bought it for speculative purposes, and when urban expansion has already pushed up the price of land on the periphery to very high levels.

Large schemes (greater than about 200 ha or with more than 500 farm units) need a full-time professional staff to manage them, and can afford to pay for it out of land rents, water charges or, where this management staff also runs the farm and employs those who work on it, from the sale of produce.

The body that manages the scheme, either by running it as a plantation or by distributing wastewater to individual farmers, is often distinct from the sanitation agency responsible for collecting and treating the wastewater. This may enable it to relate more closely to the Ministry of Agriculture or of Water Resources and may give it greater freedom of action, which can be advantageous given the uncertainties of weather and agricultural prices; on the other hand, its lack of control over treatment means that it is dependent on good relations with another agency for the reliable implementation of what is usually the principal measure for health protection.

In some of the most efficient schemes (for instance, at Werribee, Australia — see Section 3.1.1), the whole operation, from collection of the wastewater, through its treatment and application, to the sale of the crop or livestock, is run by a single agency. Where this is not possible, some local arrangement for intersectoral coordination will be needed, as at national or regional level (see Section 8.1.2). It is particularly important that the areas of responsibility of each relevant agency should be clearly defined.

A common measure, particularly in schemes using wastewater from a public sewerage network, is to issue permits for the use of the resource. These are usually issued by the local agriculture or water resources administration, or by the body controlling the wastewater distribution system. Provision for such permits is often made in the existing water resources legislation to control abstraction, but when wastes are to be used the issuing and renewal of a permit can be made conditional on the observance of sanitary practices regarding application methods, crop restriction and exposure control. A permit system can also be applied to the use of excreta, especially where the excreta is collected by a municipal body, and to aquaculture.

It is also common for the body administering the distribution of wastewater to deal with the farmers or pond owners through users' associations, which will often develop from traditional institutions.

Permits to use the wastes can then be issued to the associations, which simplifies the administrative task of dealing separately with a large number of small users and also delegates to the associations the task of enforcing the regulations which must be complied with for a permit to be renewed.

A joint committee or management board, which may include representatives of these associations, as well as any particularly large users, the authorities that collect and distribute the wastes, and also the local health authorities, is another institution which has proved its worth in many schemes, for example in Calcutta (see Box 8.9). Even in small-scale organizations, some arrangement such as a committee with community representatives is essential for the users to participate in the management of the project.

Box 8.9 Management of wastewater use in Calcutta

Wastewater from Calcutta is conveyed to the wetlands east of the city through two main canals, from which it passes into a complex system of secondary and tertiary channels. From these, a regulated amount is fed into an extensive system of ponds through simple gates; the fishermen have learned over the years how to judge the amount needed by taste, smell and sight.

There are some 160 owners of ponds in the area, most of whom are absentee landlords working through resident managers. Each employs from 50 to 200 fishermen, mostly on a seasonal basis, and owns up to 400 ha. Some have leased the land from the Calcutta city authorities, and there are also three fishermen's cooperatives with their own ponds. Altogether about 4000 families live by fishing in some 5000 ha of pond area.

Some of the wastewater is used to irrigate vegetables grown on the nearby garbage dump where some 2000 families farm 1400 ha. Lease of this land was granted in 1879 by the city authorities but is currently under dispute; a three-tier pattern of ownership now exists, with lessees letting out the garbage gardens to tenants who in turn receive payment from farm workers.

Further downstream, wastewater treated in the pond system is used to irrigate approximately 6500 ha of paddy fields, from which 5000 families earn all or part of their income.

A joint committee, comprising pond-owners, downstream land-owners and Calcutta city authorities, has recently been set up to deal with problems of common concern such as irregularities in the supply of sewage and theft of fish by armed gangs!

Source: Strauss (1986d).

Further details of wastewater use in Calcutta are given in Section 3.

Support services

Various support services to farmers are particularly relevant to the implementation of health protection measures, and detailed consideration should be given to them at the planning stage. They include the following:

- farm machinery (sales and servicing, or hire);

- supply of supplementary fertilizers, irrigation pipe, protective clothing, etc.;

- agricultural credit;

- agricultural extension and training;

- marketing services, especially where new crops are to be introduced or new land brought into productive use;

- primary health care, possibly including regular health checks for field workers and their families (see Section 7.5).

Training

Training requirements must be carefully evaluated at the planning stage, and it may often be necessary to start training programmes, especially for farmers and operators, before the project begins, in order to ensure that an adequately trained cadre is available when needed. Plant operators require on-the-job training in all aspects of the operation of treatment plant, delivery systems and pumping stations, farmers will need training in agronomic methods most suitable for excreta and wastewater use, and technicians will require training in sample collection and analysis.

Similarly the likely need for agricultural and aquacultural extension services must be estimated, and provision made for them to be available to farmers after implementation of the project. Extension officers will themselves need training in the farming methods appropriate to health protection, as will the staff responsible for enforcing sanitary regulations regarding crop restriction, occupational health, food hygiene, etc.

Such training requirements are best met by local technical colleges and universities, but many countries may lack the specific expertise needed; overseas training may then be the only alternative in the short term until sufficient in-country experience is developed. This is an area in which cooperation between neighbouring countries can be especially fruitful.

8.3.5 Legislation

If new projects for the use of wastewater or excreta for agriculture or aquaculture are to be introduced or promoted, legislative action may be needed. In many cases it may be sufficient to amend existing regulations, but sometimes new legislation is required. Five areas deserve attention:

- creation of new institutions or allocation of new powers to existing bodies;

- roles of and relationships between national and local government in the sector;

- rights of access to and ownership of wastes, including public regulation of their use;

- land tenure;

- public health and agricultural legislation: waste quality standards, crop restrictions, application methods, occupational health, food hygiene, etc.

These are discussed in turn.

Creation of new institutions

Enabling legislation may be required to establish a national co-ordinating body for the sector (see Section 8.1.2) and to set up local bodies to manage individual schemes. These will require a certain degree of autonomy from central government and the ability either to charge for the wastes they distribute or to sell any crops they produce.

National and local government

The local body managing a scheme, or at least the agency collecting the wastes, will often be under municipal control. If new schemes are to be promoted in the context of a national policy, this implies careful coordination and definition of the relationship between local and national government. On the one hand, it may be necessary for the national government to offer incentives to local authorities to promote new schemes, but at the same time, sanctions of some sort may have to be applied to ensure that schemes are implemented without undue risk to public health.

Incentives may take the form of grants, low-interest loans or technical assistance for the establishment of new schemes. Another incentive, with possible application in arid areas, is to offer increased rights of abstraction of surface or ground water for water supply development to municipalities that develop wastewater irrigation (see Box 8.10). Sanctions might be needed to ensure compliance by municipal wastewater treatment works with national wastewater quality standards; if no such legislation exists, consideration should be given to enacting it in the broader context of environmental pollution control.

Rights of access

Farmers will be reluctant to install irrigation infrastructure, to build fish-ponds, etc. unless they have some confidence that they will continue to have access to the wastes. On the other hand, this access may be regulated by permits and dependent on efficient or sanitary practice by the farmer. In Mexico, the authorities' power to withhold water from farmers who do not comply with crop restrictions is a major factor in their success. In Chile, on the other hand, the water law vests water rights in the owners of the land, and the sanitary authorities have little leverage to impose much-needed restrictions (Bartone & Arlosoroff, 1987). Legislation may therefore be required to define the users' rights of access to the wastes and the powers of those entitled to allocate or regulate those rights.

Land tenure

Security of access to wastes is worth little without security of land tenure. Existing land tenure legislation is likely to be adequate for most eventualities, although it may be necessary to define the ownership of virgin land newly brought under cultivation. If it is decided to amalgamate individual farms under a single management, powers of compulsory purchase may be needed.

Public health

The area of public health includes rules governing crop restrictions and methods of application, as well as quality standards for treated

Box 8.10 Mexican national programme for wastewater use

The National Programme for the Use of Wastewater in Mexico is being set up to answer the increasing demand for water — by agriculture, industry and domestic users. The basis of the programme is that clean water, in areas where it is used for irrigation or in industry, can be 'exchanged' with wastewater, thereby releasing the clean water for domestic use while satisfying the water demands of agriculture and industry. In addition, using wastewater instead of disposing of it in rivers will reduce the level of environmental contamination and contribute to pollution control. The programme is currently in the planning stage, and final decisions on its execution have not yet been made.

At present, most of the untreated wastewater from large- and medium-sized cities is used for irrigation and six organized irrigation district units completely depend on this source of irrigation water. A total of 2400 million cubic metres of wastewater is used per year to irrigate 156 000 ha of land. It is planned to increase this to an annual 2600 million cubic metres of wastewater on 237 000 ha of land in 17 irrigation districts in 6 states. In this way, first-use water will be freed to supply the domestic and industrial water demand of 29 million inhabitants.

The planning of this programme will involve state and municipal governments, as well as industrial concerns, coordinated by the Ministry of Agriculture and Water Resources (SARH) which has the power to allocate water rights. It is likely that the sewage from each municipality will need some form of treatment before it can be used in agriculture. Regulations for the use of wastewater will be drawn up through coordination between SARH (including the Sub-Secretariat of Agriculture) and the Ministry of Urban Development and Ecology with the support of the World Health Organization. If the wastewater does not meet the regulations, SARH will demand that the municipality involved must treat it to the specified quality before it is 'exchanged' with the clean water. SARH will advise on the most appropriate type of treatment via a coordinated group of ministries, including the Ministry of Urban Development and Ecology and the Ministry of Health. Help with the finance needed to effect this treatment will be given by the Ministry of Urban Development and Ecology.

Source: H. Romero, personal communication.

wastewater and excreta used in agriculture or aquaculture, which may require an addition to existing regulations. It also covers other aspects of health protection, such as occupational health and food hygiene, which are unlikely to need any new measures. The risk of passing laws that are too stringent to be realistically complied with is just as significant with new schemes as in the case of an existing practice (see Section 8.2.2). The factors affecting the feasibility of enforcing crop restrictions, discussed in Section 8.2.3, are equally relevant to new schemes.

8.3.6 Public relations and information

The maintenance of good public relations, especially with respect to protection of consumer health, is a very important task. The public must have confidence that the produce they are consuming is in no way injurious to their health. Schemes for excreta and wastewater use must be seen by the public to be operated with due regard for their health, and assurances as to the quality of the food consumed and of the efficacy of excreta and wastewater treatment prior to land or pond application will do much to promote public acceptance of such schemes. In this respect, programmes for the routine monitoring of excreta and wastewater and of crop quality are extremely important, as is the demonstrated absence of the transmission of excreta-related disease (see Section 8.5).

The public should be kept informed about all schemes for excreta and wastewater use—whether agricultural or aquacultural, including tree and green space irrigation or land reclamation—so that they may fully appreciate governmental efforts to improve food supplies, safeguard health and protect the environment. The choice of communications media—for example newspapers, posters, radio—should be made with due regard to local customs and advertising practice, as it is important that public information campaigns about excreta and wastewater use produce the correct impact at reasonable cost.

The consumer need not be the only target of public information activity. Current and potential users of the waste and owners of (and workers in) the fields or ponds where wastes can be used must be informed of the potential for increased production and of the measures needed to safeguard health. Health education is essential where human exposure control is part of the health protection strategy. Promotional activity and health education are more effective when carried out through people in the community than through mass media. However, this requires a considerable number of dedicated staff, unless it can be achieved through an existing network of community workers.

8.4 Economic and financial considerations

Economic factors are especially important when the viability of a new scheme for the use of wastewater or excreta is being appraised, but even an economically worthwhile project can founder without careful financial planning. Economic appraisal considers whether a project is worth while, whereas financial planning looks at how projects are to be paid for. Improvements to existing practices must be paid for in some way and therefore also require some financial planning. The two areas are discussed in turn.

8.4.1 Economic appraisal

The economic appraisal of an excreta or wastewater use project is undertaken to determine the advisability, in relation to the country's economy, of proceeding with it (Squire & van der Tak, 1975; Gittinger, 1982), and thus seeks to answer the question of whether the country can afford it. This requires a calculation of the marginal costs and benefits of the project, that is, the differences between the costs and benefits of the project and the costs and benefits of the alternative. For a scheme to be viable, its marginal benefits must exceed its marginal costs.

Wastewater

The economic appraisal of wastewater irrigation schemes is compli-cated by the fact that the alternative—what would be done in the absence of the scheme—might be any of the following:

• no agriculture at all;

• no irrigation at all (that is, rain-fed agriculture);

• irrigation with water from an alternative source without fertilizer application; or

• irrigation with water from an alternative source with fertilizer application.

The marginal benefit accruing from wastewater irrigation is different in each case.

Where land is a scarce resource, the objective may be to obtain the maximum marginal benefit per hectare. In other cases, especially those where the alternative is no agriculture at all, the most significantly scarce resource is water, and the aim is to obtain the greatest benefit from every cubic metre of wastewater used. The appraisal of a specific project involves not only comparing it with all the appropriate alternatives but also comparing possible variants of the same scheme — for instance, the use of different irrigation methods or the production of different crops.

The cost of the wastewater includes the cost of any additional treatment required (to bring it to the Engelberg standard for instance), as well as the cost of conveying it to the field and applying it to the crop. However, it is essential to subtract from this the cost of the alternative arrangements for wastewater disposal which would be required if the project were not implemented. Thus, if the alternative would involve some treatment, only the cost of additional treatment would be included.

In many cases, the alternative involves expensive long-distance transport of wastes or sea outfalls, so that reuse may be the cheapest disposal option even before the value of agricultural production is included. This rationale justifies the use of wastewater to irrigate municipal parks and gardens, as in some cities in the Eastern Mediterranean area and the USA.

If the alternative is to be rain-fed agriculture or irrigation with fresh water from another source, the values of the alternative crop yields and the costs of any fertilizer used must be taken into account. One particular benefit of wastewater irrigation is the saving in the cost of abstracting fresh water from its source — especially when that fresh water might otherwise be valuable for such purposes as industrial and domestic supplies. Unfortunately, it is often the case that insufficient information is available to allow the full costs and benefits of the alternative to be calculated, and wastewater use must then be compared with the alternative of no irrigation at all or, more commonly, of no agriculture.

Economic appraisal recognizes that the real cost or value of an item to a country's economy is not always the same as the price paid for it. For example, foreign exchange may in fact be more valuable than the formal, controlled exchange rate would suggest. On the other hand, the labour of workers who would otherwise be unemployed costs less to the economy than their wages, since no production is lost elsewhere by offering them a job. Economists use a 'shadow price' to approximate the 'real' value of an item to the national economy. Thus the shadow price of foreign exchange is usually higher, and that of unskilled labour lower, than the rate actually paid for it.

The use of shadow prices is particularly important for the economic appraisal of wastewater use schemes, and tends to favour them for at least two reasons. First, the treatment process most appropriate for wastewater irrigation (stabilization ponds) can be built by labour-intensive methods and requires less imported equipment than other processes; at shadow prices, it is more likely to be cheaper. Second, the prices of many of the crops likely to be grown in a scheme (such as cereals, oilseeds and cotton) are often held below the world market price. Whether they are grown for export or for import substitution, a shadow price for foreign exchange will show their true value to the economy.

Excreta

Methods for the economic appraisal of excreta use schemes are less sophisticated than those for wastewater irrigation, since some of the benefits — such as improvement of the soil structure — are much more difficult to quantify. The alternative is taken to be one of no fertilization at all, and thus an excreta use scheme would be judged to be economically viable solely if the value of its resulting marginal benefit (increased crop yield) were greater than the cost of excreta treatment, conveyance and application.

Aquaculture

There are two possible alternatives for comparison:

* no aquaculture at all;

* aquaculture with an alternative source of pond fertilizer.

Economic appraisal is thus similar to that of wastewater irrigation, and a viable benefit-cost ratio implies that the marginal value of the fish or aquatic crops produced is greater than the cost of the treatment and conveyance of the excreta or wastewater used to produce them.

8.4.2 Financial planning

Charging for the resource

Where wastewater is distributed by a separate agency from that which collects and treats it, a charge of some sort is normally payable.

Charges are also levied when the waste is distributed to individual farmers.

The level of these charges must be decided at the planning stage (see Box 8.11). The Government must decide whether they should be set to cover only the operation and maintenance costs or set higher to recover the capital costs of the scheme as well. While it is of course desirable to ensure the maximum recovery of costs, an important consideration is to avoid discouraging the farmers from the permitted use of the wastes. Some prior investigation of farmers' willingness and ability to pay is therefore essential, not only in determining the level of charges but also the frequency, time and means of payment. For instance, an annual charge payable after the harvest season may be the easiest to collect.

Box 8.11 Wastewater reuse in Trujillo, Peru

Trujillo is a city of 400 000 inhabitants situated on the arid north-central coast of Peru. An existing sewer system serves almost 90% of the population, discharging directly on to the beach just to the north of the urbanized area. However, wastewater is extracted at several points for authorized sugar-cane or forage crop irrigation, and at several other points clandestine derivations are made by local farmers for food crop irrigation. In some cases, farmers have constructed rudimentary pond systems to treat the wastewater in order to obtain irrigation "permits", but these ponds are in fact nothing more than shallow anaerobic settling basins with retention times of about one day. The economic demand for irrigation water is great, as there is no rainfall throughout the year and a nearby river has streamflow for only five months of the year. Large areas of barren desert land that surround Trujillo could be put into agricultural production if water were available.

As part of a feasibility study done for the National Water and Sewerage Service with the financial support of the German agency Gesellschaft für Technische Zusammenarbeit, a planned effluent irrigation option was evaluated. It was found that of a total of 2100 ha suitable for irrigation, only 1300 ha could be irrigated throughout the year with the available wastewater volume (approximately 20.5 million cubic metres per year in 1990). By dividing the existing sewer system into micro-drainage areas it was possible to identify eight points in the system where wastewater could be diverted for gravity-fed irrigation after treatment in appropriately designed waste stabilization ponds. The chemical characteristics of the wastewater presented no problem for irrigation, so the principal concern was pathogen removal for which multicell ponds provide a good solution.

163

> **(Box 8.11 continued)**
>
> A financial analysis of the proposed reuse scheme with and without treatment showed that irrigation with treated wastewater would be feasible only if there was a fair allocation of the treatment costs between the principal beneficiaries — that is, between the municipality, which needs to dispose of its wastewaters in a sanitary manner, and the farmers who require irrigation water of adequate quality. The cost allocation formula recommended for Trujillo was to charge the construction costs to the municipality and the land costs and operation and maintenance costs to the farmers. A survey of local farmers found that they were agreeable to cost-sharing at this level in the form of either water tariffs or in-kind contributions of land and labour (a finding substantiated by the fact that some farmers were currently using ground water at about twice the cost allocated to them for treated wastewater). Using this formula, the reuse project is financially viable.
>
> This example illustrates the fact that local farmers are often able and willing to pay for the effluents they use for irrigation, but that they should not be expected to subsidize the legitimate disposal costs of the municipality.
>
> *Source:* Rojas et al. (1985).

It may be possible to develop an increased demand for the wastes by effective marketing, and this will often be worth while. However, the results of a marketing campaign should not be anticipated when setting the initial level of charges, which can be increased progressively as demand is developed.

On the other hand, farmers may sometimes be willing to share in the investment in treatment works that are a prerequisite to obtaining reuse permits. Their contribution may be in cash or in the form of land for treatment or storage facilities. Moreover, experiences in Peru have indicated that farmers may sometimes be willing to perform operational and maintenance tasks associated with treatment, storage and conveyance of wastes, as a contribution in kind to the running costs of the scheme (Bartone & Arlosoroff, 1987).

A farmer will pay for wastewater to irrigate crops only if its cost is less than that of the cheapest alternative water and the value of the nutrients that it contains. How then is the cost of the wastewater determined by the agency that sells it to the farmer? There are three basic approaches to establishing the price of wastewater. It can be related to:

- its production costs (additional treatment and conveyance);

- the benefits derived from irrigation; or

- some value judgement based on the farmers' ability or willingness to pay.

If the first option is selected, it should carry the proviso that costs must be no greater than that of the cheapest alternative source of water available to the farmers (usually ground water). The nutrient value of the wastewater may be included or ignored.

In the case of aquaculture and the use of excreta in agriculture, the price for the excreta or wastewater is usually based either on the marginal cost of treatment and conveyance or on the value of the nutrient (usually nitrogen) content, whichever is lower. There are several possible ways of charging for the waste, such as:

- per cubic metre (or, for excreta, per ton);

- per hour of discharge from a standard sluice;

- per hectare of irrigated or fertilized land.

It can also be paid in various ways:

- as a specific water rate or purchase price;

- as a renewal fee for an abstraction permit;

- as a surcharge on the land rent;

- as a deduction from the price of centrally marketed crops.

A particular problem needing prior consideration is the question of liability and the action to be taken when, for one reason or another (for example, because of a breakdown in the treatment works), the wastes do not meet the agreed quality requirements. It will be difficult to prevent farmers from using the wastes, particularly if this happens at a time of peak demand when the lack of water or fertilizer could seriously prejudice plant growth. The simplest solution is probably to exempt the farmers from charges for the period when the wastes fail to meet the quality standard. They should of course be informed of the problem and the health risks involved, and every possible temporary measure should be taken to keep those risks to a minimum until normal quality is restored.

Payment for health protection

It is not always appropriate or feasible to meet the cost of health protection by charging for the use of the wastes. Financial considerations regarding each of the four types of health protection measure are discussed below.

(a) Treatment

Wastewater. Wastewater treatment works are expensive to build; the heavy capital investment required exceeds the resources of most municipalities in developing countries, so it is usually met, together with the cost of the sewerage system, by grants or loans from central government. The operating costs, on the other hand, can usually be met from a municipal tax or water tariff. The costs of treatment are usually justified on grounds of environmental pollution control.

However, the treatment of wastewater to a standard of quality adequate for use in agriculture may involve additional costs for construction and maintenance. Some of these additional costs can be met by the sale of the treated wastewater or the fee for the permit allowing its use. In practice, however, the prices charged for the wastewater and the fees levied for permits are often determined by what farmers are prepared to pay. In such cases, the difference may be considered as a government subsidy to the farmers to promote the use of the wastewater. It is common in practice for irrigation water to be supplied to farmers at subsidized rates.

Excreta. The capital cost of nightsoil treatment can be very modest and part, at least, of the treatment cost can be recovered from the sale of the treated nightsoil. It is likely to consist largely of recurrent operating costs and to be relatively small in comparison with the cost of collecting the raw excreta. If the market value of the treated product is low, the balance of the treatment cost can be met from the same budget that supports the nightsoil collection service. This may even represent a saving in relation to the greater alternative cost of disposing of the untreated excreta. When the excreta are composted together with domestic refuse, the saving in the cost of disposing of solid waste can be considerable.

If individual farmers are to be encouraged to treat nightsoil or wastewater, for instance by building a nightsoil storage tank or — in the case of aquaculture — by separating off part of a fish-pond, they may need credit to help them with the capital cost of any construction required. An existing agricultural credit system can be used to implement this, if it can give specific priority to farmers using wastes.

(b) Crop restriction

The demands of crop restriction for the purpose of health protection often run against the incentives of the market; salad vegetables, for example, are often more profitable than industrial crops. A farmer who complies with crop restriction regulations that prohibit salad crops will thus make less money than one who disobeys them. The difference in profit is the cost of compliance. To some extent this cost is a result of market distortions, because the prices of the crops carrying a smaller health risk (such as cotton, grains and oilseeds) are often kept artificially low by the government or by marketing boards. At uncontrolled prices, such as the world market prices, some of these crops might be almost as profitable as the crops forbidden by the regulations. Their production may be as valuable to the national economy, although the farmer is paid less for them. In these circumstances, it would be perfectly rational for the government to subsidize the use of wastes, subject to crop restrictions, as a correction to the price distortion.

However, it is not usually feasible to pay this subsidy in the form of a higher price for the permitted crops. A two-tier price system (a subsidized price for the crop when grown using wastes, and a lower price otherwise) would be open to abuse; on the other hand it is not a simple matter to remove existing price distortions that affect the country as a whole. The subsidy can be paid more easily in the form of government support for other measures, particularly health protection measures involving treatment and application of wastes and human exposure control.

Nevertheless, these other forms of subsidy will not remove a price incentive to the farmer to disobey crop restrictions. The regulations have to be enforced, and this also costs money. The enforcement is normally carried out by the body that issues permits to use the wastes (often the Ministry of Agriculture) or by local staff of the Ministry of Health. In either case, enforcement of crop restrictions is only one of many tasks performed by the staff responsible, so the cost is usually included in the budget that supports their salaries, transport, etc. However, this is not an excuse for neglecting the cost of establishing an efficient enforcement system. Crop restriction may mean that less need be spent on treatment, but it will not be effective if adequate financial provision is not made for its enforcement.

(c) Application

Sprinkler irrigation, which potentially causes more widespread contamination with wastewater than other methods, generally requires less preparation of the land than surface irrigation. If surface or subsurface irrigation is chosen to minimize this contamination, the land can often be prepared more easily and cheaply by a central organization than by individual farmers. Alternatively, farmers can be assisted with the loan or hire of the necessary equipment. Since preparation of the fields helps the farmers avoid other expenditure, the cost can be recovered from them in the same way as other irrigation costs — through land rent, water charges or permit fees. Since localized irrigation uses less water and can produce higher yields, farmers themselves may find it worth while to change to this method.

(d) Human exposure control

The purchase of protective clothing will normally be at the expense of the workers who wear it or of their employers.

It might be possible for the cost of regular treatment for intestinal helminths to be charged to large employers, for example by a surcharge on the fees they pay for a permit to use wastewater. However, if the treatment is carried out by the national health service, the procedure for reimbursing the Health Ministry for the cost of the treatment from a fee paid to another body may be complicated. It is not advisable to charge the farmers for the treatment, as chemotherapy should be free if full coverage is to be attained. The cost is therefore likely to be most conveniently borne by the normal budget of the health service.

8.5 Monitoring and evaluation

The combination of health protection measures adopted in a particular wastes reuse scheme is a complex system that requires regular monitoring to ensure that it continues to function effectively. Monitoring, however, in the sense of observing, inspecting and collecting samples for analysis, is not sufficient on its own. Institutional arrangements must be made for the information collected in this way to provide feedback to those who implement the health protection measures. In other words, answers must be provided in advance to the following questions:

(a) What information will be collected?

(b) How often and by whom?

(c) To whom will this monitoring information be given?

(d) What decisions will be taken on the basis of the monitoring information?

(e) What powers will exist to ensure that those decisions are implemented?

To answer question (d) requires a set of guidelines or standards with which the monitoring results can be compared. There are two types of answer to question (e). First, in the case of monitoring by an operating agency (for instance a municipal sewerage board), those who interpret the monitoring information can simply give orders to their subordinates to take any corrective action needed. Second, in the case of surveillance by an enforcement agency (for instance a Ministry of Health), the agency has legal powers to enforce compliance with quality standards and other legislation. A complete monitoring and control system therefore needs:

• guidelines or standards;

• monitoring or surveillance to assess compliance;

• institutional arrangements for feedback or enforcement.

The responsibility for the monitoring of health protection measures must be clearly defined at the outset if it is not to be neglected. Appropriate aspects for regular monitoring and evaluation include the following:

• implementation of the measures themselves;

- microbiological quality of the wastes;

- microbiological quality of the crops;

- surveillance of disease in exposed groups.

Implementation of the measures

The principal health protection measure in many cases will be treatment of the wastes to adequate standards of quality (see below). The implementation of the other measures can be monitored by surveys as described for existing practices in Section 8.2.1. These need to be conducted at more frequent intervals during the first months of operation of a new scheme, but the frequency can be progressively reduced to once or twice a year once any initial problems have been ironed out.

Wastes quality

With regard to wastes treatment, it may be more fruitful to monitor the functioning of the treatment system than to take frequent samples of the treated waste for microbiological analysis, which can be difficult, time-consuming and expensive. Monitoring of the hydraulic loading on a set of stabilization ponds, for instance, is relatively easy and can immediately explain any deterioration in effluent quality which would be inexplicable on the basis of micro-biological data alone.

In particular, the Engelberg guideline values are not intended as standards for quality surveillance but as design goals to be used when planning a treatment system.

Nevertheless, the agency responsible for the operation of the larger nightsoil or wastewater treatment works should carry out a regular check on the microbiological quality of the treated wastes, at least for faecal coliforms. In many cases, however, the only body with the necessary laboratory facilities for a full microbiological examination is the Ministry of Health or the local health administration. Whether or not it carries out the laboratory tests for the wastes treatment agency, the Health Ministry is usually best placed to maintain overall surveillance of the quality of wastes used in agriculture and aquaculture. For surveillance purposes, the samples for examination should be collected, as well as examined, by the government department responsible, to ensure that the results are interpreted in true perspective.

Since intestinal nematodes are a major health risk, and their eggs are more persistent than faecal bacteria, it would be ideal if the laboratory examination were to include a test for the concentration of intestinal nematode eggs. However, the laboratory techniques involved are still at an experimental stage.

Samples should be collected under aseptic procedures and examined within 6 hours of collection. Between collection and bacteriological examination they should be kept at about 4 °C, for instance on ice in an insulated coolbox. Where the effluent has been disinfected with chlorine, samples should be dechlorinated immediately and special care taken to prevent the regrowth of bacteria. Field testing will be more appropriate in many cases than transportation to a laboratory. Samples should preferably be collected by staff of the laboratory where they will be examined. If this is not possible, particular attention must be paid to proper sample identification and presentation; details of bacteriological test procedures are given elsewhere (American Public Health Association, 1985). A simplified procedure for faecal coliform bacteria is described in Box 8.12.

A procedure for enumerating nematode eggs in wastewater samples is given in Box 8.13; for excreta samples the formol-saline-ether method may be used (Cheesbrough & McArthur, 1976). Note that nematode eggs are usually removed but not killed by sedimentation in wastewater treatment, whereas in the treatment of excreta they are usually killed but not removed. Thus in wastewater examination it is not necessary to ascertain whether the eggs are viable, whereas this is the primary concern when examining samples of excreta.

Samples of treated excreta and wastewater should be taken at least monthly for physicochemical analyses — pH, electrical conductivity, sodium adsorption ratio, nutrients (N, P, K) and boron — although this frequency may be relaxed if experience shows that the quality variation is small. Heavy metals should be included in the analysis if the wastewater contains a significant proportion of industrial waste.

Large excreta or wastewater use schemes may warrant the establishment of their own laboratory facilities for these analyses, but existing laboratories will generally be used. Local hospitals usually have facilities for microbiological analyses, and the chemical analyses may be done at local wastewater treatment works, schools or colleges, although for some analyses samples may need to be sent to a central laboratory (for example, the Laboratory of the Government Chemist or equivalent). However, lack of local laboratory capacity for quality monitoring is not an adequate reason for failing to make use of wastes.

Box 8.12   Simplified analysis for faecal coliforms

This procedure tests whether or not wastewater meets the Engelberg guideline of 1000 faecal coliforms per 100 ml for unrestricted irrigation.

Use normal aseptic procedures throughout. Prepare a 1 in 10 dilution by adding 1 ml of the wastewater sample to 9 ml of 8.5 g/l (0.85%) sodium chloride solution. Add 1 ml of diluted sample to each of 5 tubes containing 5 ml of A-1 medium[a] and a Durham tube. Incubate at 44.5 °C for 19–23 h. Count the number of positive tubes (those showing gas production), and read the most probable number (MPN) of faecal coliforms per 100 ml of wastewater from the following table.

Number of positive tubes	MPN of faecal coliforms per 100 ml
0	<220
1	220
2	510
3	920
4	1600
5	>1600

Use the same procedure for samples of treated nightsoil. Shake the sample thoroughly and add 1 ml (or 1 g) to a screwcapped bottle containing 9 ml of diluent and a few glass beads. Shake the diluted sample thoroughly before adding to the tubes of A-1 medium.

[a] Composition: lactose, 5 g; tryptone, 20 g; NaCl, 5 g; Triton X-100, 1 ml; distilled water, 1 litre (American Public Health Association, 1985).

Crop quality

Monitoring of the microbiological quality of crops is also likely to be the responsibility of the Ministry of Health in its role as enforcer of the existing public health regulations. Where fodder crops are involved, this task will include the inspection for beef and pork tapeworm of the carcasses of animals fed with (or grazed on) these crops. Inspection should cover *all* carcasses and not just a sample. All infected carcasses should be rejected.

Box 8.13 Quantitative determination of helminth eggs in wastewater

This method, adapted from Teichmann (1986), relies on centrifugal flotation.

Procedure

1. Grab-samples of at least 1 litre of wastewater should be taken at a fixed time of day for each site and transported to the laboratory.

2. In the laboratory each sample is placed in a 1-litre beaker (15 cm diameter) and allowed to settle for 8 hours. Sedimentation can occur overnight and the procedure be continued the next day.

3. After sedimentation the supernatant is removed by using a water jet (vacuum) pump.

4. The sediment is transferred into 20-ml centrifuge tubes (maximum 3 ml per tube). The walls of the sedimentation beaker should be cleaned thoroughly using a spray bottle and the rinsing water added to the sediments in the centrifuge tubes. They are then centrifuged for 10 minutes at 700g and the supernatants are discarded.

5. 3 ml of $NaNO_3$ solution (500 g/l) are added to the sediment in each tube. The sodium nitrate solution should have a relative density of 1.3 (*Note*: if the relative density is too low, the centrifugal flotation will not work properly and some eggs will not float to the surface).

6. After adding $NaNO_3$, the tubes are centrifuged for 3 minutes at 1000g.

7. The supernatant (now containing the helminth eggs) is removed carefully and kept in a 1-litre beaker (15 cm diameter) containing just less than 1 litre of pure water. (The water dilutes the sodium nitrate so that the eggs will settle to the bottom of the beaker.)

8. 3 ml of $NaNO_3$ solution are again added to the sediment in each tube, and the tubes are centrifuged at 1000g for 3 minutes. The supernatant is carefully removed and added to the 1-litre beaker containing the first supernatant.

9. The procedure in (8) is repeated (so that the sediment is centrifuged with sodium nitrate a total of three times).

(Box 8.13 continued)

10. The beaker containing all the supernatants diluted in water is left for several hours, to allow all the helminth eggs to settle to the bottom.

11. The supernatant from this beaker is carefully removed and discarded, and the sediment is transferred to centrifuge tubes. The walls of the sedimentation beaker should be cleaned thoroughly using a spray bottle, and the rinsing water added to the sediment in the centrifuge tubes. The tubes are then centrifuged for 4 minutes at 1000g.

12. The final centrifugate is placed on slides and examined under the microscope. It can be brightened up with paraffin oil after evaporation of the water. Helminth egg counts are made under × 100 magnification.

Variants

- Instead of collecting all the supernatants from the sodium nitrate centrifugation in a beaker of water for resedimentation, the supernatants from all three centrifugations (steps 6 to 9) can be filtered through a membrane filter (pore diameter approximately 10 μm). The filters can be air-dried in neutral balm embedded on slides or they can be viewed directly and egg counts made. Use of membrane filtration is probably simpler and more efficient, but also more costly, than the above procedure.

- In steps 2 and 7, the 1-litre beaker can be replaced by a 1-litre conical flask. This will encourage sedimentation and may produce a higher recovery rate of eggs. Use of several smaller conical containers (such as urine flasks) could be considered.

- If sodium nitrate is not available, magnesium sulfate of a similar relative density could be tried. The percentage recovery with MgSO$_4$ has, however, not been assessed.

Recovery rate

Using this procedure, recovery is about 70%, when egg density is 100 per litre. When the egg density decreases, the recovery rate also decreases. At 10 eggs per litre, recovery is about 50% and at 1 egg per litre it is further reduced to 33%.

Disease surveillance

Disease surveillance should focus first upon farm workers, who are the group most likely to be exposed to infection as a result of using wastewater or excreta. The simplest form of surveillance, and therefore the minimum for any waste reuse scheme, is a regular stool survey of a sample of workers for intestinal parasites. This is best carried out at a fixed time of year, because of the tendency to seasonal variation in the prevalence and intensity of infection with several of these parasites. If chemotherapy is administered, a survey can conveniently be carried out just before the annual round of treatment.

Surveillance of diarrhoeal diseases poses greater difficulties; it should preferably concentrate on individual pathogens, although this is not easy. Bactèriological examination of stools is expensive and may not give very consistent results. However, where typhoid is endemic, a serological survey using the Widal test (Cheesbrough & McArthur, 1976) would be relatively easy to carry out at the same time as the collection of stool samples for the parasitological survey.

The epidemiological considerations (sample size, ethics, interpretation of results and so on) that are relevant to disease surveillance are very similar to those that should govern an epidemiological survey (see Box 8.3). An epidemiologist and a statistician should be involved in planning the surveillance programme, and should also be consulted if any apparent excess disease is detected among exposed groups of people.

References

ANON. Processing sludge and manure. *Biocycle*, **27**(2): 30–31 (1986).

AMERICAN PUBLIC HEALTH ASSOCIATION. *Standard methods for the examination of water and wastewater*, 16th ed. New York, American Public Health Association, 1985.

ARTHUR, J. P. *Notes on the design and operation of waste stabilization ponds in warm climates of developing countries*. Washington, DC, World Bank, 1983 (Technical Paper No. 7).

AYERS, R. S. & WESTCOT, D. W. *Water quality for agriculture*. Rome, Food and Agriculture Organization of the United Nations, 1984 (Irrigation and Drainage Paper No. 29, Rev. 1).

BARTONE, C. R. ET AL. *Monitoring and maintenance of treated water quality in the San Juan lagoons supporting aquaculture*. Lima, Pan American Center for Sanitary Engineering and Environmental Sciences, 1985.

BARTONE, C. R. & ARLOSOROFF, S. Reuse of pond effluents in developing countries. *Water science and technology*, **19**(12): 289–297 (1987).

BLUM, D. & FEACHEM, R. G. *Health aspects of nightsoil and sludge use in agriculture and aquaculture. Part III: An epidemiological perspective*. Dübendorf, International Reference Centre for Waste Disposal, 1985 (Report No. 05/85).

BOSE, P. C. Calcutta sewage and fish culture. *Proceedings of the National Institute of Sciences of India*, **10**(4): 443–454 (1944).

BURAS, N. ET AL. Microbiological aspects of fish grown in treated wastewater. *Water research*, **21**: 1–10 (1987).

CACERES, A. & CACERES, R. *Control sanitario de bio-anobos y efluentes de letrinas secas familiares y digestores de biogas*. Unpublished paper presented at XIII Congresso Centroamericano de Ingegnieria Sanitaria y Ambiental, Guatemala City, Guatemala, 16–20 March 1981.

CALIFORNIA STATE DEPARTMENT OF PUBLIC HEALTH. *Statewide standards for the safe direct use of reclaimed wastewater for irrigation and recreational impoundments*. Berkeley, California State Department of Public Health, 1968 (California Administrative Code, Title 17 — Public Health).

CAMP SCOTT FURPHY PTY LTD. *Werribee treatment complex development strategy. Stage 1 Report — Report to the Melbourne and Metropolitan Board of Works*. Melbourne, Camp Scott Furphy Pty Ltd, 1986.

CHAO, K. *Agricultural production in communist China* (1949–1965). Madison, University of Wisconsin Press, 1970.

CHAMBERS, C. W. Chlorination for control of bacteria and viruses in treatment plant effluents. *Journal of the Water Pollution Control Federation*, 43: 228–241 (1971).

CHEESBROUGH, M. & MCARTHUR, J. *A laboratory manual for rural tropical hospitals*. Edinburgh, Churchill Livingstone, 1976.

CROSS, P. *Health aspects of nightsoil and sludge use in agriculture and aquaculture. Part I: Existing practices and beliefs in the utilization of human excreta*. Dübendorf, International Reference Centre for Waste Disposal, 1985 (Report No. 04/85).

COUNCIL OF THE EUROPEAN COMMUNITIES. Council Directive 76/160/EEE of 8 December 1975 concerning the quality of bathing water. *Official journal of the European Communities*, L31: 1–7 (5 February 1976).

COWAN, J. P. & JOHNSON, P. R. Reuse of sewage for agriculture in the Middle East. In: *Reuse of sewage effluent*. London, Thomas Telford, 1985, pp. 107–127.

DONEEN, L. D. & WESTCOT, D. W. *Irrigation practice and management*. Rome, Food and Agriculture Organization of the United Nations, 1984 (Irrigation and Drainage Paper No. 1, Rev. 1).

DURON, N. S. Mexican experience in using sewage effluent for large-scale irrigation. In: Pescod, M. B. & Arar, A., ed. *Proceedings of the FAO Regional Seminar on the Treatment and Use of Sewage Effluent for Irrigation, Nicosia, 7–9 October 1985*. London, Butterworths, 1985.

EDWARDS, P. *Aquaculture: a component of low-cost sanitation technology*. Washington, DC, World Bank, 1985 (Technical Paper No. 26).

EDWARDS, P. & KAEWPAITOON, K. *Fish culture for small-scale farmers*. Bangkok, Environment Sanitation Information Center, Asian Institute of Technology, 1984.

FAO. *China: recycling of organic wastes in agriculture*. Rome, Food and Agriculture Organization of the United Nations, 1977 (Soils Bulletin No. 40).

FAROOQ, S. & ANSARI, Z. I. Water reuse in Muslim countries — an Islamic perspective. *Environmental management*, 7 (2): 119–123 (1983).

FEACHEM, R. G. ET AL. *Sanitation and disease: health aspects of excreta and wastewater management. World Bank Studies in Water Supply and Sanitation 3*. Chichester, John Wiley, 1983.

FLEISS, J. L. *Statistical methods for rates and proportions*, 2nd ed. Chichester, John Wiley, 1981.

FORDHAM, J. W. Development of wastewater reuse programmes. In: *Intercountry Seminar on Wastewater Reuse, Manama, 29 September– 2 October 1984.* Unpublished document WHO-EM/ES/351 of the WHO Regional Office for the Eastern Mediterranean.

GAMBRILL, M. P. ET AL. Microcomputer-aided design of waste stabilization ponds in tourist areas of Mediterranean Europe. *The public health engineer*, 14 (2): 39–41 (1986).

GITTINGER, J. P. *Economic analysis of agricultural projects*. Baltimore, Johns Hopkins University Press, 1982.

GOTAAS, H. B. *Sanitary disposal and reclamation of organic wastes*. Geneva, World Health Organization, 1956. (Monograph Series No. 31).

HILLEL, D. *The efficient use of water in irrigation: principles and practices for improving irrigation in arid and semiarid regions.* Washington, DC, World Bank, 1987 (Technical Paper No. 64).

HUGGINS, R. J. Constructive use of sewage with regard to fisheries. In: *Reuse of sewage effluent.* London, Thomas Telford, 1985, pp. 147–155.

INTERNATIONAL REFERENCE CENTRE FOR WASTE DISPOSAL. Health aspects of wastewater and excreta use in agriculture and aquaculture: the Engelberg report. *IRCWD news*, **23**: 11–18 (1985).

KAYSER, R. The use of biologically treated wastewater together with excess sludge for irrigation. In: Pescod, M. B. & Arar, A., ed. *Proceedings of the FAO Regional Seminar on the Treatment and Use of Sewage Effluent for Irrigation, Nicosia, 7–9 October 1985.* London, Butterworths, 1985.

KING, F. H. *Farmers of forty centuries*. London, Jonathan Cape, 1926.

KIRBY, C. F. Irrigation with wastewater at Board of Works Farm, Werribee. In: *Water on the farm.* Report No. 25, Kingsford, NSW, Water Research Foundation of Australia, 1967, pp. 37–41.

KRISHNAMOORTHI, K. P. ET AL. Intestinal parasitic infections associated with sewage farm workers with special reference to helminths and protozoa. In: Saraf, R. K., ed. *Proceedings of the Symposium on Environmental Pollution, Nagpur, India.* Central Public Health Engineering Research Institute, 1973, pp. 347–355.

LEWIS, W. J. ET AL. *The risk of groundwater pollution by on-site sanitation in developing countries.* Dübendorf, International Reference Centre for Waste Disposal, 1982 (Report No. 01/82).

LWANGA, S. K. & LEMESHOW, S. *Sample size determination in health studies.* Geneva, World Health Organization, in press.

MARA, D. D. *Sewage treatment in hot climates.* Chichester, John Wiley, 1976.

MARA, D. D. ET AL. Brazilian stabilization pond research suggests low-cost urban applications. *World water,* **6** (7): 20–24 (1983).

MARA, D. D. & SILVA, S. A. Removal of intestinal nematode eggs in tropical waste stabilization ponds. *Journal of tropical medicine and hygiene,* **89** (2): 71–74 (1986).

MARA, D. D. ET AL. The performance of a series of five deep ponds in northeast Brazil. *Water science and technology,* **19** (12): 61–64 (1987).

MEADOWS, B. S. Fish production in waste stabilization ponds. In: Cotton, A. & Pickford, J., ed. *Sanitation and water for development in Africa.* Loughborough, WEDC Group, University of Technology, 1983, pp. 39–42.

ORAGUI, J. I. ET AL. The removal of excreted bacteria and viruses in deep waste stabilization ponds in northeast Brazil. *Water science and technology,* **19** (12): 569–573 (1987).

ORON, G. ET AL. Effluent in trickle irrigation of cotton in arid zones. *Journal of the Irrigation and Drainage Division, American Society of Civil Engineers,* **108** (IR2): 115–126 (1982).

OTIS, R. J. & MARA, D. D. *The design of small-bore sewer systems.* Washington, DC, World Bank, 1985 (TAG Technical Note No. 14).

PAYNE, A. J. The use of sewage waste in warm water agriculture. In: *Reuse of sewage effluent.* London, Thomas Telford, 1985, pp. 157–171.

PEREIRA NETO, J. T. ET AL. Pathogen survival in a refuse/sludge forced aeration compost system. In: *Effluent treatment and disposal,* Oxford, Pergamon Press, 1986, pp. 373–391.

PEREIRA NETO, J. T. ET AL. Low-cost controlled composting of refuse and sewage sludge. *Water science and technology,* **19** (12): 839–845 (1987).

PETTYGROVE, G. S. & ASANO, T. *Irrigation with reclaimed municipal wastewater — a guidance manual.* Sacramento, California State Water Resources Board, 1984 (Report No. 84–1).

POLPRASERT, C. ET AL. *Recycling rural and urban nightsoil in Thailand.* Bangkok, Asian Institute of Technology, 1982.

ROJAS, R. ET AL. *Tratamiento y disposición final de las aguas servidas de Trujillo.* Lima, CEPIS, 1985.

ROMERO, H. *Wastewater use in agriculture in developing countries: how crop control can be used as a sanitary controlling measure.* Unpublished paper presented at Second Project Meeting on the Safe Use of Human Waste in Agriculture and Aquaculture, Adelboden, Switzerland, 15–19 June 1987.

RYDZEWSKI, J. R. *Irrigation development planning: an introduction for engineers.* Chichester, John Wiley, 1987.

SAGARDOY, J. A. *Organization, operation and maintenance of irrigation schemes.* Rome, Food and Agriculture Organization of the United Nations, 1982 (Irrigation and Drainage Paper No. 40).

SHENDE, G. B. Status of wastewater treatment and agricultural reuse with special reference to Indian experience and research and development needs. In: Pescod, M. B. & Arar, A., ed. *Proceedings of the FAO Regional Seminar on the Treatment and Use of Sewage Effluent for Irrigation, Nicosia, 7–9 October 1985.* London, Butterworths, 1985.

SHUVAL, H. I. ET AL. *Wastewater irrigation in developing countries: health effects and technical solutions.* Washington, DC, World Bank, 1986 (Technical Paper No. 51).

SIMPSON-HEBERT, M. *Methods for gathering socio-cultural data for water supply and sanitation projects.* Washington, DC, World Bank, 1983 (TAG Technical Note No. 1).

SQUIRE, L. & VAN DER TAK, H. G. *Economic analysis of projects.* Baltimore, Johns Hopkins University Press, 1975.

STENTIFORD, E. I. & PEREIRA NETO, J. T. Simplified system for refuse/sludge composting. *Biocycle,* **26** (5): 46–49 (1985).

STRAUSS, M. Survival of excreted pathogens in excreta and faecal sludges. *IRCWD news,* **23**: 4–9 (1985).

STRAUSS, M. *About agricultural use of wastewater and excreta in Latin America.* Dübendorf, International Reference Centre for Waste Disposal, 1986a.

STRAUSS, M. *Wastewater use in Tunisia.* Dübendorf, International Reference Centre for Waste Disposal, 1986b.

STRAUSS, M. *Excreta disposal and fish culture in Indonesia.* Dübendorf, International Reference Centre for Waste Disposal, 1986c.

STRAUSS, M. *Wastewater and excreta use in India.* Dübendorf, International Centre for Waste Disposal, 1986d.

STRAUSS, M. *Notes on the reuse practice in selected countries of the Gulf region, northern Africa and Latin America.* Unpublished paper presented at the Seminar on Effluent Reuse, Ministry of Health, Oman, April 1987.

TAPIADOR, D. D. ET AL. *Freshwater fisheries and aquaculture in China*. Rome, Food and Agriculture Organization of the United Nations, 1977 (Fisheries Technical Paper No. 168).

TEICHMANN, A. Zur Methodik des quantitaven Nachweises von Helminthenstadien in kommunalen Abwässern. *Angewandte Parasitologie*, 27: 145–150 (1986).

UNITED NATIONS CENTRE FOR HUMAN SETTLEMENTS. *The design of shallow sewer systems*. Nairobi, United Nations Centre for Human Settlements, 1987.

VENUGOPALAN, V. Foreword. In: Roy, A. K. et al., ed. *Manual on the design, construction and maintenance of low-cost waterseal latrines in India*. Washington, DC, World Bank, 1984 (TAG Technical Note No. 10).

VILLALOBOS, G. G. ET AL. Program for the reuse of wastewater in Mexico City. In: D'Itri, F. M. et al., ed. *Municipal wastewater in agriculture*. New York, Academic Press, 1981, pp. 105–144.

WATER AUTHORITIES ASSOCIATION. *Waterfacts*. London, Water Authorities Association, 1985.

WATER RESEARCH CENTRE. *Disinfection of sewage by chlorination*. Stevenage, Water Research Centre, 1979 (Notes on Water Research No. 23).

WATER RESEARCH CENTRE. *Application of sewage sludge to agricultural land*: *a directory of equipment*. Medmenham, Water Research Centre, 1984.

WOHLFARTH, G. Utilization of manure in fishfarming. In: Pastakia, C. M., ed. *Fishfarming and wastes*. London, Janssen Services, 1978, pp. 78–91.

WORLD HEALTH ORGANIZATION. *Reuse of effluents: methods of wastewater treatment and health safeguards*; report of a WHO Meeting of Experts. Geneva, WHO, 1973 (Technical Report Series No. 517).

WORLD HEALTH ORGANIZATION. *The risk to health of microbes in sewage sludge applied to land*. Copenhagen, WHO Regional Office for Europe, 1981a (EURO Reports and Studies No. 54).

WORLD HEALTH ORGANIZATION. *Manual for the planning and evaluation of national diarrhoeal diseases control programmes*. Geneva, WHO, 1981b (WHO/CDD/SER/81.5).

WORLD HEALTH ORGANIZATION. *Guidelines on studies in environmental health*. Geneva, WHO, 1983 (Environmental Health Criteria 27).

WORLD HEALTH ORGANIZATION. *Guidelines for drinking-water quality. Volume 1. Recommendations*. Geneva, WHO, 1984.

WORLD HEALTH ORGANIZATION. *Health guidelines for the use of wastewater in agriculture and aquaculture*: report of a WHO Scientific Group. Geneva, WHO, 1989 (Technical Report Series No. 778).

ZANDSTRA, I. *Reclamation of nutrients, water and energy from wastes: a review of selected IDRC-supported research*. Ottawa, International Development Research Centre, 1986 (Manuscript Report No. IDRC-MR124e).

ZHONGJIE, Z. Treatment and reuse of human wastes, and the present state of water resources, in China. *Water science and technology*, 18 (6/7): 9–12 (1986).

Bibliography

This Bibliography is not an exhaustive list of documents on the subject of human wastes reuse, but it includes many of the major recent sources in the field and will thus serve as a useful lead-in to the literature. Consideration has also been given to the availability and ease of acquisition of these works in developing countries. Many other useful documents are listed in the References section.

ANON. Reuse of sewage effluent. In: *Proceedings of the International Symposium organized by the Institution of Civil Engineers, London, 30–31 October 1984.* London, Thomas Telford, 1985.

ARAR, A. & PESCOD, M. B. *Treatment and use of sewage effluent for irrigation.* Sevenoaks, Butterworth, 1987.

DALZELL, H. W. ET AL. *Soil management: compost production and use in tropical and subtropical environments.* Rome, Food and Agriculture Organization of the United Nations, 1987 (Soils Bulletin, No. 56).

D'ITRI, F. M. ET AL. *Municipal wastewater in agriculture.* New York, Academic Press, 1981.

FINKEL, H. J. *Handbook of irrigation technology, Vols 1 and 2.* Boca Raton, CRC Press, 1983.

McGARRY, M. G. & STAINFORTH, J. *Compost, fertilizer and biogas production from human and farm wastes in the People's Republic of China.* Ottawa, International Development Research Centre, 1978.

OBENG, L. A. & WRIGHT, F. W. *The co-composting of domestic solid and human wastes.* Washington, DC, World Bank, 1987.

SHUVAL, H. I. *Water renovation and reuse.* New York, Academic Press, 1977.

SHUVAL, H. I. *Water quality management under conditions of scarcity: Israel as a casestudy.* New York, Academic Press, 1980.

STRAUSS, M. *Health aspects of nightsoil and sludge use in agriculture and aquaculture. Part II: Pathogen survival.* Dübendorf, International Reference Centre for Waste Disposal, 1985 (Report No. 04/85).

UNITED NATIONS ECONOMIC AND SOCIAL COMMISSION FOR WESTERN ASIA. *Wastewater reuse and its application in Western Asia.* Baghdad, UN-ESCWA, 1985.

Glossary

Note. Words <u>underlined</u> are also explained in this glossary.

biofiltration A <u>conventional treatment</u> process for wastewater, also known as the trickling filter, in which the <u>wastewater</u> trickles through a well ventilated bed of coarse material.

BOD Biochemical oxygen demand, a measure of the amount of organic matter in <u>wastewater</u>.

burden The number of parasitic worms with which a person is infected. This is also called the intensity of infection.

compost The humus-like product of the decomposition of excreta mixed with organic material rich in carbon.

depuration The practice of transferring fish to an unfertilized pond for a short period before harvesting.

desludge Remove accumulated <u>sludge</u> from septic tanks, etc.

ditch, oxidation A channel, also known as the Pasveer ditch, in which <u>wastewater</u> circulates in the course of the treatment process and is aerated by a large rotor.

dose, infectious The number of pathogens ·that· must simultaneously enter the body, on average, to cause infection.

effluent Outflowing liquid. Treated effluent flows out from a <u>wastewater</u> treatment plant.

emitter The small aperture from which water is applied to each plant in <u>localized irrigation</u>.

eutrophication The enrichment of natural waters, especially by compounds of nitrogen and phosphorus, resulting in increased productivity of some species of plants.

evapotranspiration The movement of water drawn up by plant roots and its evaporation from leaves and the soil.

excreta Faeces and urine. In these Guidelines the term is used also to refer to <u>sludge</u>, <u>septage</u> and <u>nightsoil</u>.

exposure control Measures taken to ensure that a <u>potential risk</u> posed by pathogens in the environment does not cause an <u>actual risk</u> of disease.

feedlot A piece of land set aside for the feeding of animals.

filter, trickling see <u>biofiltration</u>.

helminth A worm; the helminths discussed in these Guidelines are parasitic worms, e.g. *Ascaris*, *Schistosoma* and *Taenia*.

hydrogeology The study of the presence and movement of water in the ground.

incidence The number of cases of a specified disease diagnosed or reported during a defined period of time, divided by the number of persons at risk in the population in which the disease occurred.

indicator organism An indicator organism is one whose presence indicates a potential risk from one or more species of pathogen.

intensity The intensity of infection with a parasitic worm is the same as the worm burden.

irrigation, border An irrigation technique by which water is admitted to the top end of a sloping strip of land and allowed to flow evenly across the full width of the strip.

irrigation, localized Irrigation by a system that applies water directly to individual plants.

lagoon, aerated An adaptation of the waste stabilization pond, in which oxygen is added by mechanical aerators.

latent The latent period of a pathogen is the time it requires to develop in the environment before it can cause infection.

latrine, pour-flush A latrine with a water seal but which can be flushed with a small amount of water poured by hand.

latrine, twin pit A form of pit latrine with two pits, which are used alternately to facilitate emptying.

leaching The draining of water through soil or other material, carrying soluble salts with it in dissolved form.

loading The loading of a wastewater treatment system is the rate at which wastewater or BOD is fed into it.

macrophyte Any plant visible to the naked eye; aquatic macrophytes float on water.

mean, geometric The mean calculated on a logarithmic scale.

mesophilic Mesophilic bacteria are those whose optimum temperature for growth is between 20 °C and 40 °C.

nematode A roundworm of the class Nematoda, e.g. *Ascaris*.

nightsoil Human excreta transported without flushing water.

phytotoxin Any substance poisonous to plants.

polyculture The production of several fish species in a single pond.

pond, facultative A pond that is aerobic near the surface but anaerobic lower down.

pond, maturation The final pond(s) in a series of waste stabilization ponds. Maturation ponds are entirely aerobic.

pond, stabilization A pond for the treatment of wastewater. Ponds are usually connected in series, with a total retention time of one or more weeks.

prevalence The number of persons sick or exhibiting a certain condition at a particular time (regardless of when that illness or condition began) divided by the number of persons at risk in the population in which it occurred.

refuse Rubbish or garbage; solid waste.

retention time The period of time wastewater takes to pass through a pond or other treatment process, calculated by dividing its volume by the flow of wastewater.

riparian Relating to the ownership of a stretch of river bank.

risk, actual Probability of an individual's developing a particular disease over a specified period.

risk, potential The chance of infection or disease that might occur but that does not at present occur.

salinization Excessive accumulation of salt.

sedimentation The process by which suspended solid particles in water or sewage are allowed to settle out to the bottom of a tank or pond.

septage Sludge removed from septic tanks.

settleable Capable of removal by sedimentation.

sewage Human excreta and wastewater, flushed along a sewer pipe.

sewer A pipe containing wastewater or sewage.

sewerage A system of sewer pipes.

sludge A mixture of solids and water deposited on the bottom of septic tanks, ponds, etc.

sludge, activated A common method of biological sewage treatment. Settled sewage is supplied either by mechanical agitation or by diffused aeration. The bacteria that grow in the medium, together with other solids, are removed as a sludge in a secondary sedimentation tank and recycled to the aeration tank inlet.

soakaway An arrangement to promote seepage of effluent into the ground.

sodicity Concentration of sodium.

sprinkler An irrigation device that applies water by spraying it over the ground.

thermophilic Thermophilic bacteria are those whose optimum temperature for growth is over 45 °C.

treatment, conventional This terms refers to the wastewater treatment processes routinely used in Europe, including biofiltration, activated sludge and oxidation ditches. The retention time of these processes is normally no more than a few hours.

trematode Flat worms of the class Trematoda, including the parasitic worms called flukes. Trematodes of medical importance have intermediate stages in snails, e.g. *Schistosoma*.

wastewater In these Guidelines, wastewater refers to the liquid waste discharged from homes, commercial premises and similar sources to individual disposal systems or to municipal sewer pipes, and consists mainly of human excreta and used water. It may contain small amounts of industrial waste, but the consequences of this are not considered in these Guidelines.

windrow A long pile of solid material undergoing composting. The pile is usually turned at intervals in order to aerate it.